Defining and Redefining EMDR

Innovative and integrative technique, diagnosis, ego states work & performance enhancement. Includes two full verbatim EMDR sessions.

DAVID GRAND, Ph.D.

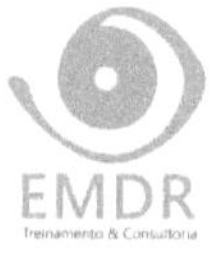

2013

Defining and Redefining EMDR

Title ID: 061587939X
ISBN-13: 978-0615879390
EMDR Treinamento e Consultoria Ltda.

www.emdrbrasil.com.br
E-mail: info@emdrbrasil.com.br

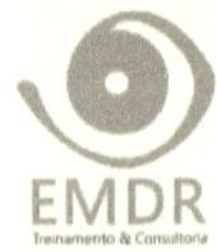

SEPS 705/905 Ed. Santa Cruz sala 441
70.390 Brasília, DF Brasil
55 61 3443 8447
www.emdrbrasil.com.br

Cover art: Esly Regina Carvalho, Ph.D.
Lay-out and editorial work: Esly Regina Carvalho, Ph.D.

This book is also available in Spanish (paperback and kindle/e-book) and Portuguese (paperback and kindle/e-book)

INTRODUCTION

What is the purpose of this book?

It is my hope to present to you in this book - innovative and integrative ideas - that will stimulate your thinking about the theory and practice of EMDR. First - a caveat - I am presenting here my ideas - that are derived from my own practice - however I want you to be exposed to different ways of practicing EMDR. I will present a variety of ideas, give my rationales - following which you should consider whatever seems to makes sense or is of interest to you. Don't try to copy anything - make the ideas your own by integrating them into how you are presently using EMDR and in terms of what fits comfortably into your personal style.

What are the EMDR basics you must learn before you can begin to redefine its practice?

It is crucial to have a full technical knowledge of EMDR before you begin to experiment with modifications of technique. It is a mistake to wander around before you know and understand the basic procedures and use of the protocol. An experienced and grounded EMDR therapist can begin to use their creative abilities to develop innovative approaches to help those who are low-responders and even apparent non-responders. Accordingly, once you have mastered the foundation you can consider incorporating your creative abilities, thus bringing EMDR to places it hasn't been before.

One of the key things in developing as an EMDR therapist is your facility with the basic technical knowledge. You must know the 8 steps and in particular the protocol inside and out. Unfortunately, many therapists complete the EMDR training afraid to use it instead of liberated by its potential. Encouragement needs to be provided to novices who forget they bring a wealth of experience to EMDR. We all have much to offer to those who suffer - as you gain experience and confidence with the basic structure of EMDR, you can make it your own in both professional and personal terms.

Are variations in EMDR practices based on personal and professional style OK?

I have observed that the EMDR trainings generally do not sufficiently address the fact that clinicians conduct therapy with different levels of variation. This also applies to EMDR, despite the clearly delineated 8 steps and the structured protocol. Accordingly, we perform EMDR in our own style - influenced by both our clinical and personal individuality. I want to support the reality that all of us use EMDR somewhat differently - as long as we operate within its basic constructs. In order to practice any therapy, especially EMDR, you need to feel comfortable and confident. No one can practice effectively while in the grips of fear. If you experience using EMDR as walking across a minefield, you can't fully utilize your resources and provide a safe, consistent holding environment for your clients.

You need encouragement to feel comfortable with the variations of approach that have derived from your individual style. Many EMDR therapists are inhibited by the fear that unless they conduct it "the right way" - it won't work or that something terrible is going to happen. Most of you are experienced, grounded therapists work prudently - as they have predating their EMDR training. These ideas are the basic tenet of his book. It bears repeating how essential it is to feel comfortable and confident - especially when challenged by the unexpected - to figure out a modification of approach on the spur of the moment - when EMDR is stalled in movement and unsuccessful in lowering the distress level.

EMDR is an experimental process - as is all therapy - you can't predict or control what happens next or the client's response to our actions. Your interventions, choice of targets, how you set up the protocol and introduce interweaves, are speculative predictors of the client's response. You act and observe the outcome. When your intervention yields and unsuccessful outcome - you have an opportunity to learn why it didn't work and take corrective measures. However, if you are fortunate enough to guess right, you may not learn why your action worked. Psychotherapy is a quintessential trial and error process.

PART ONE - DEFINING

What do you mean by "Defining and Redefining EMDR?"

The act of determining a target and identifying it in the aspects of the protocol (image, cognition, affect and body sensations) is a psychologically and neurologically defining process. Combined with the bilateral activation (eye movements, auditory or tactile stimulation) this defining produces the rapid, direct movement observed and resolution obtained in EMDR processing.

Both working with complex cases and developing applications beyond trauma work such as performance enhancement, call for a redefining of EMDR beyond the basic structure taught in the Level I and II Trainings. The themes of innovation and integration are interwoven throughout this book.

Most of the technical innovations in this book can be categorized as advanced interweaves. The term "cognitive interweave" is a limited one. Many forms of interweaves exist - for example - highlighting body sensations, affects, sensory experience and ego states which also can activate stalled processing. Most novices don't realize how technical EMDR is as it can appear so straightforward. Seasoned therapists usually experience the more they practice EMDR, the more they realize how complex it is. As you learn - you will encounter the ever-expanding vista of how much there is to know. It is important to pursue individual and group supervision for guidance by experienced EMDR experts - who should also be pursuing their own learning process. At this developmental stage as an EMDR therapist - I am learning more than I have at any prior point - in fact I am experiencing an acceleration process!

Defining and redefining EMDR connotes expanded and varied ways of conceptualizing and working with the protocol. In the situation where the client naturally processes without blocking or looping - usually when the target is a discrete trauma or a simple phobia - then less need arises to include modifications. These are the situations where processing flows steadily and naturally - when you stop the client periodically to ask, "Where did you go with that," - and observe ongoing movement. The process continues until the client desensitizes to a zero SUDS and installs the PC to a seven VOC. How often have you found that EMDR proceeds in this fashion? This is reminiscent of when we were children - no told how difficult life in the adult world was going to be - until we discovered it on our own. When originally trained in EMDR I don't recall being informed that most cases were going to be complex. Accordingly, as I began practicing I was confused, frightened and discouraged. I thought that I was no doing it correctly or that EMDR is effective with most of the people who come to us for help - although modifications and more sessions than were originally expected are needed.

Certain clients need preparatory work before we can respond effectively to EMDR. You can be traumatized by targeting a discrete trauma that doesn't process through as it is perched upon significant childhood trauma and dissociative defenses ("you mean the DES and history taking doesn't always pick it up?"). Application of EMDR has powerfully demonstrated the ubiquity of profound trauma and dissociative defenses. This phenomenon requires us to develop and integrate with EMDR a spectrum of advanced techniques (interweaves) to make a successful treatment possible. Considerable attention will be addressed in this book to these approaches.

A defining question - What is and what isn't EMDR?

The questions has been raised, "What is and what isn't EMDR?" My opinion is that EMDR occurs when you identify a target with the client - define it by the protocol, (image, cognition, affect and body sensation) and then apply the bilateral stimulation which activates accelerated information processing (mind movement). This process accomplishes shift and hopefully resolution of what has coalesced within the target. Yet, within these boundaries considerable latitude exists. However, I believe bilateral stimulation without a defined target does not constitute EMDR. It is also not EMDR if you construct a protocol and don't activate it with bilateral stimulation. Each of these approaches may be effective ways of addressing certain situations - but it is the two together which produce the EMDR effect.

If treatment is conducted with either bilateral auditory or tactile stimulation running constantly - following the determination of the protocol - including in between sets, is this EMDR? Although this is nontraditional, it still qualifies as EMDR. However, what if a target and a protocol are no determined and the stimulation is present in this unstructured format? This might be designated as a derivative of EMDR. Would the use of part of the protocol - perhaps only body sensations with bilateral stimulation - constitute EMDR? This remains a debatable point.

Francine Shapiro has clearly stated that eye movements alone are not EMDR. It is in combination with the eight steps of preparation and application of the protocol (comprised of the target defined and rated as image, cognitions, affect and body sensations). This is the clearest definition to date. However, many additions have been made to this process which has made the picture less clear.

Firstly, the predominance of eye movements as the sole or even primary mode of bilateral stimulation has shifted. Francine discovered EMDR with eye movements (perhaps the tactile aspect of walking also contributed) which continues to be the main mode taught in the trainings - until recently auditory and tactile bilateral activation were presented as secondary.

The development of the cognitive interweave (CI) and the future template have opened the gates to innovative and integrative interweaves. The CI was originally intended to be introduced when a client was blocked or looping - to help guide past the points of resistance. With the recognition that most cases we treat are complex - the concept of interweave naturally was expanded to integrate the vast wealth of technical knowledge and experiential wisdom sourcing from EMDR therapists prior training and clinical exposure. Ego State work is an example of advanced interweaving applied to make the EMDR feasible or more effective. If it is subsumed under the protocol, then this advanced interweave certainly falls under the rubric of EMDR.

What is the scope of EMDR?

Our techniques are not solutions - they are tools. The solution is held in the client's neurophysiological capacity to heal and our belief in and feel for his process.

With some regularity a client has come to me reporting that a previous EMDR therapist has told her/him, EMDR doesn't work with your situation." Often it is patently obvious that the person will likely respond favorably to EMDR. Other clients present challenges requiring technical modifications or an extended time frame with EMDR. Either the prior therapist was lacking in experience or knowledge or perhaps was unconsciously afraid of opening up the client's intensely traumatic material.

Why should we "assume nothing" with EMDR? How does this relate to educating our clients?

One of my guiding principles in EMDR is "ASSUME NOTING". In our pre-EMDR lives as therapists we relied upon assumptions - otherwise we had no organized basis from which to understand or intervene. In contrast - EMDR is truly client-centered - the true answers lie only within the individual. Accordingly, our assumptions tend to interfere with the emergence of the client's truth(s). The therapy process is not only one that we must continually learn and relearn - the same educational dynamic applies to our clients' experience. Ergo, fully educating the client in the EMDR process is crucial and exceeds the informing process of most other therapies.

A good example of the client's need to acquire knowledge about the process is exemplified when they report "nothing happened" (the EMDR therapist's nightmare). I take issue with the first response we are taught in trainings - the instruction to change the direction of the eye movement. This is usually a technical mistake - could "nothing" really happen? Usually something did happen but the client didn't recognize it. If we don't explore it with them - they will miss an opportunity to gain knowledge about the nature of EMDR processing. In fact, these impasses are wonderful opportunities to educate the client. When a client finishes a set and reports, "nothing happened" try asking, "Let me check something out with you. You started with this image - where did you immediately go next?" sometimes the client answers, "It disappeared, nothing happened." This indicates that the client was unaware very powerful and rapid processing actually occurred. Another client might report, "I just started to think about something else, nothing happened." You might hear, "My mind started to jump around to all kinds of different places, nothing happened," or "I started to think about something from the distant past, nothing happened." When you accept these erroneous beliefs that "nothing happened" and instruct them to change the direction of eye movements, you are reinforcing an incorrect notion as well as missing an opportunity to educate the client.

How can we tell if the client is processing effectively?

Some clients experience obscure and/or strange processing such as seeing colors, flashing lights or cartoon images. How do you - as well as your clients - determine if this is effective processing or not? The best approach is to return the client to target and see if the image looks and feels any different, if the affect or body sensations have changed and you observe if there is any shift in the SUDS level. Even, if it has risen, processing is happening.

In EMDR you start by setting up the basic structure - the target defined by the protocol. Within this structure, when you introduce an interweave you narrow the focus of the processing - both informationally and neurologically. It can be speculated that an effective interweave activates movement when processing has stalled. Accordingly, we can conceptualize working with interweaves - within the protocol - as defining, redefining, narrowing down, reactivation - followed by re-expanding back to the full protocol. With certain clients it is necessary to maintain a narrowed focus for a longer period of time with more therapist involvement (active interweaving) to initiate and sustain movement.

How do you form an effective negative cognition with high functioning clients?

Question: Many of my clients are high functioning and spiritually oriented. They are reluctant to say something negative about themselves in the present, i.e., "I am not good enough;" "I deserve only bad things," "I am permanently damaged," etc. How do you form a workable NC with those who are hesitant to say negative things about themselves in the present? In other words, they have no problem saying, "I was inadequate, worthless, helpless, powerless at the time of the trauma" - but not in present time. I sometimes process the NC in the past tense, and when it desensitizes they are able to come up with an appropriate PC in present time. I know that's not the usual procedure, but there are times when it appears that's all I have to work with.

Answer: This goes to a new EMDR interest of mine - understanding the wide variation of communication, semantics and thinking styles we encounter with our clients. These phenomena are often subtly intertwined with the cultural differences our clients present. Often we erroneously assume we fully comprehend words or meanings when we do not. An abiding credo of mine in EMDR is "ASSUME NOTHING!"

It is relevant to note that as you practice in the mid-south. The differences from New York - where I practice - are as profound as with another country, or example attitudes, pace of life, foods (see "My Cousin Vinny" - how long do you cook a grit?), social interchange, religious beliefs and practices and very much so accents, meanings and communication patterns.

The formation of a workable negative cognition is based on our clearly communicating to (educating) the client what the NC is - and what its purpose is. Absent of that, troubles may arise later that can appear to be the process not working. You must also be careful that the client is not subtly coerced into selecting a neat NC that meets a "book" criterion but does not connect with their essential, organic beliefs. The spiritual or highly developed clients who "know better" do not escape distorted thinking, even if they are able to override their irrationality more easily than others. Unless they don't possess unconscious minds with primary process thinking at its core, it is through the educating process they you guide them to locate the irrational beliefs that unceasingly battle to escape their netherworld.

1. Think of the NC as the voice of the inner critic - who doesn't have one or even a team of them? Who doesn't in a moment of frustration say or think to themselves, "How could you be so stupid?" or "Fool, you did it again."
2. Consider the NC as a belief held by a young child-self who tends to personalize external events, particularly critical or

abusive communications from parents and other significant adult figures.

3. Remember that trauma restricts the brain's (or areas within it's) ability to process information accurately. This results in erroneous mental explanations attempting to make sense and provide a locus of control in confronting the inexplicable. "It was my fault" or "I'm bad" are two such examples.

4. Unless these beliefs are identified, they may block - or at least not be worked through - in the EMDR processing.

5. Statements that don't appear to fit the criteria of the NC may confuse us. Upon further exploration I have discovered that "I was out of control," "I feel bad," "I don't know," "Why," among others were in the client's lexicon, acceptable as NCs and at times their core negative belief. Ferreting out detective work is one of your primary clinical skills.

6. How you communicate the purpose and meaning of the NC is critical. "What strange or distorted beliefs still remain in the dark recesses of your mind that pop out at you, even though you know they are not true?" "If you close your eyes and put yourself back in the situation, what negative beliefs come up now?"

If a NC cannot be elicited when forming the protocol, it can be deferred and will often emerge later. However, a target issue or memory can resolve even if we never overtly define the NC. You may assume that it was imbedded in the experience and was swept away without ever showing itself outright.

Is "It's my fault" an acceptable negative cognition?

Can someone please explain why "It's my fault" is not a preferred self-referencing negative cognition? I have had several molestation victims use this NC and it seemed to work well. But in recent discussions I heard with some facilitators it was pointed out that it isn't self-referencing and therefore can't be processed properly. Does it depend on the type of trauma experienced or does it leave the client open to some responsibility which they may interpret as blame and thereby not be able to reach the core belief?

Answer: In relation to the NC - "It's my fault" - it appears to me to be very serviceable - and your results verify it. The only exception would be when a person was in reality at fault, such as a drunk driver or a perpetrator. There may be cases where a more core NC would be elicited if you asked the client, "if it is (was) your fault, what does that lead you to believe about yourself, now?" This aims uncovering more global or pernicious beliefs i.e. "I deserve to be punished," "I am worthless," "I am bad," "I suck," "I am a terrible person," "I am dirty," "I am unlovable," etc. however, NCs should not be "prepackaged" or externally imposed to fit a standard. Language is so individualized that at times a statement that technically seems totally unusable such as "I felt sad" or "Not now" may, in the client's lexicon, be the best representation of their negative, distorted self-belief in the present. This is consistent with the context of EMDR as client-centered and defined. It remains our task to respectfully and assiduously determine what the client's words semantically express for them.

What is "EMDR Diagnosis?"

EMDR can serve as a valuable diagnostic tool. When you carefully attend to your client's processing, you discover a wealth of information you might not discover otherwise - and you receive validation or invalidation of your hypotheses. In other words - the accelerated information processing of EMDR often yields heretofore inaccessible information on the mental processes and personal history of the client. This can rapidly provide the therapist with an accurate and comprehensive diagnostic picture that might not otherwise emerge well into the treatment process, if at all. EMDR is particularly helpful in diagnosing anxiety disorders, bi-polar and affective conditions, dissociative disorders, character pathology, somatoform and pain syndromes, addictions and co-dependency, as well as identifying areas of strength, healthy development and resiliency. Another ego psychological approach is the diagnostic practice of developmental blueprinting. This approach is characterized by identifying lesions (or blockages) as well as areas of health on the developmental lines of separation/individuation, defense mechanisms, anxiety level and super-ego functioning.

Another example of diagnostic EMDR pertains to body sensations. Observing the nature of what occurs during the processing of the body sensations yields considerable information. Have you witnessed somatic sensations originating in one location, moving to another, and continuing to travel without processing out, despite material emerging? With which diagnostic condition is body fluxing usually associated? I have found a high correlation between sensate movement and anxiety conditions - frequently panic disorders. When you already know that a client has a panic disorder - this is a way to confirm the diagnosis. When you don't know - body fluxing indicates that an underlying panic disorder may be present.

On the other hand - when a body sensation doesn't move or change - it suggests an organic basis to the symptom as opposed to emotional derived. Always make sure that your clients are fully checked out medically. Occasionally you will treat a person suffering from gastric burning for many years and the symptom processes through in one session and it's gone! At other times EMDR results in partial change and in other situation nothing shifts. On occasion these symptoms will disappear and return an hour, a day or a week later. These all constitute meaningful diagnostic indicators. Firstly, it helps determine whether the symptom is organic or psychogenic in basis. Secondly, if it is psychogenic, you need to determine its derivation(s). Clients with completely blocked processing, are likely responding to the activation of the threatened breakout or early trauma associated with terror. A memory that evokes extreme anxiety states may unconsciously feel safer to keep locked away in perpetuity.

At times EMDR processing results in glacial movement - the client starts at a SUDS of 8 and ends the session at a 7.89. This very slow movement is usually a diagnostic indicator of characterological problems or a dissociative condition that doesn't explode out with processing. When movement is painfully slow you need to examine, review and ask yourself, "Have I looked at the characterological aspects of the individual?" "Have I looked in the history and determined how it developed?" "Can I observe any other manifestations of character pathology, narcissism, explosiveness, sociopathy - the tendency to project issues outward?" This can be a diagnostic indicator or a guide towards locating some dissociative defenses that is buried underneath - slowing or undermining the response to the process.

What is the Questioning Interweave?

The "questioning interweave" is an effective technique in redirecting the client's questions as well as a way of forming non-directive inquiries which effectively evoke the client's truths. Clients at times emerge from a set and ask, "Why is that so?" When this occurs how do you respond? A helpful thing to say is "ask yourself that question and go with that". When clients process questions redirected to themselves - they activate their internally held answers. And when this transpires they often recognize and observe spontaneously, "I know what the answer is!" and frequently it's not what you anticipate their answer might be. None of us are prescient enough to know in what part of a client's brain their answers are stored or what part of their memory holds their associations and solutions. At times it is helpful for you to form non-leading open-ended questions for clients can ask themselves and process. As an example, "ask yourself why you moved from this thought to the next one" or "you were processing about your accident when your thoughts shifted to summer camp."

When clients redirect questions to themselves - they are activating information stored in the brain. The subsequent processing tends to accelerate the uncovering and connecting process. I have observed remarkable responses to this approach that has direct application to dream analysis, as well. When a client brings a dream to session or retrieves a dream while processing - try posing this question to be processed: "What do you think your dream meant?" Frequently a person will observe quickly, "I know what it is!" The same approach can be applied with slips of the tongue, or when a client forgets or blocks on information. Encourage them to "Ask yourself - why did I block on that?" This is another tool to help clients make connections - applying bilateral stimulation in this way can shorten the time required or even make possible uncovering and reprocessing of significant issues.

What are some issues of Theory and Practice I should be aware of?

In EMDR training, it is taught that the protocol is completed when the SUDS level has been desensitized to a zero or one. However, stopping the sets prematurely may leave important unexplored areas or unwarranted levels of disturbance. In my experience, this is especially the case in the extended treatments where each drop of a numerical notch represents the bridging of a wide chasm. For some clients, this final step in protocol from one to zero poses the greatest challenge and may be essential for true resolution. Accordingly, the significance of the differential between zero and one should be carefully assessed on a case specific basis before moving ahead to the next phase of treatment.

Another technical innovation approach is repeated returns to target. This can facilitate overcoming impasses or accelerating crawling activity. Following each set of eye movements, the usual opportunity is provided for reflection. The client is then instructed to return to the image and negative cognition, even if processing has resumed. Varied numbers of repetitions are employed after each application. It has been my observation that four to six of these returns to target often serves as an approach that effectively reactivates a meaningful flow of associations.

Although EMDR is a highly client-centered process, you must understand when to assert yourself as issues of technical importance arise. In these situations, a thorough educational process is essential to guide and empower the client. This included the assessment of readiness for termination of treatment. Additionally before finishing a treatment, I recommend briefly reassessing all previously completed protocols to determine if they have remained fully reprocessed. Any targets with SUDS levels which have climbed back over zero, or VOCs which have dropped below seven, should be reprocessed to a point of full resolution. When all previous issues have remained fully reworked, discussions of finishing therapy are in order. EMDR clinicians should not assume that the client's attainment of emotional integration, symptom elimination and an improved level of functioning are sufficient criteria to immediately conclude treatment. The essential aspect in therapy is the relationship itself. This healing environment exists apart from the defined objectives and goals of the process. The timing of the separation from this human bond should be mutually negotiated and handled with sensitivity and attunement. The corrective experience of determining the conclusion of therapy is both required and deserved by people who have suffered the total loss of choice and control entailed in their histories of severe trauma.

People with character or personality disorders as well as those manifesting dissociative disorders - especially distinct alter states - will usually require many sessions to work through the first in depth protocol. Anticipate investing many weeks - if not many months to attain completion of the protocol. A technical error to avoid is assuming the process is not working and look for another protocol or worse to give up on using EMDR altogether with the client. As long as you observe processing - or "mind movement" as I like to call it - don't be discouraged by how slowly the SUDS level is dropping. If you persevere - your client will; be encouraged to continue and potentially obtain profound change - even full resolution - with issues tracing back to repeated early traumatization. Of course, dissociative and character disorders are not pure diagnoses - you'll often see elements of both mixed together.

People with dissociative disorders usually have suffered repeated early trauma, often mental, physical or sexual abuse. When it traces back very early - especially to a pre verbal level - it can move very slowly. Of course in working with people with dissociative disorders, you should orchestrate a full program to ensure they have the kind of support network that they need. It is essential to continue working with the protocol until it is fully completed. Applying this issue of technique, when your client returns their follow-up session, you instruct him/her to return to the target protocol. Start by saying, "If you bring up the image - what does it look like to you now?" If your client responds, "I don't want to work on that - I'm in a completely different place now. I want to work on something that happened to me this week." Acceding to this request is a technical mistake as it short-circuits the client's opportunity to fully resolve the extant protocol and its inherent conflicts. Remember to stay with a protocol until it is fully resolved - whether it takes one minute, one session, two sessions, twenty sessions, or a hundred sessions. Staying with the protocol means going back to the original target image, when starting each session. If you persevere, clients with character pathology and dissociative disorders, are able to desensitize the initial protocol down to 0 SUDS. Often times processing down from a SUDS of 2 or 1 to a 0, especially on the first protocol, is the most challenging task. When a client with a profound long-term history of trauma arrives at a 0, they have accomplished a breakthrough previously beyond their grasp. You are then ready to proceed to another protocol that will tend to process more quickly than the first one. If the initial one required six months, this one will likely take three to five months to work through. By that point you will likely understand and accept how gradually some clients process.

As their ego strengths develop - clients will process protocols more quickly and efficiently. They may proceed ahead along developmental lines and diagnostically shift into more adaptive symptoms, beliefs and behaviors. It is rewarding and profound experience to guide a client with dissociative or characterological features toward resolution. This eventually leads to communications such as, "you know something, I feel like I'm almost ready to stop!" Before EMDR, it was assumed that with clients manifesting these pathologies that the optimal goal was modification with limitations. It was beyond our scope to help them beyond a certain point. The fact that you can now - given sufficient time to use EMDR - attain full resolution is phenomenal. I have experienced this - to date - with five clients that I have treated with longer term EMDR.

Question: Can you treat clients at risk of retraumatization?

My clients live here in Northern Israel with the realistic appraisal that there may well be rocket attacks, but the actual chance of being hit or injured is much less than, say being mugged in New York. Both depend on not walking around at the wrong place or time. Of course, safety rules are paramount and they have to be instilled first. Then, if the client wishes to continue living here, as most do, the next thing that is needed is to develop a sense of proportion of the actual danger. I use EMDR as one of the ways of helping the client assess the situation in the light of what she has gone through. No doubt EMDR would ideally be used in totally calm circumstances - after an even was in the past - but we don't have that luxury. We must constantly work with the engine running. So, I agree that in some cases, I might have to go further back to earlier trauma to improve results.

Answer: You have - in my estimation - quite accurately assessed the clinical picture here and it can be categorized as EMDR remediation. I call this approach, "Calculating the Percentages." Following almost any discrete trauma (car accident, mugging, dog attack) the fear of reoccurrence is one of the primary PTSD symptoms. As Clinicians, we cannot honestly communicate that it won't happen again, but we can help our clients to better define likelihood in numerical terms.

You can start my asking - in the same manner that we elicit the distorted Negative Cognition - "What do you feel the chances are right now that you will reexperience this incident in the next week, month, year, five years?" Follow with "How often has this happened to you in the past?" (the reality template). As these questions are incorporated into the protocol and the processing, you return periodically to the first question to determine if any shift towards a more realistic assessment of percentages has occurred. Install any positive movement and continue until both you and the client agree that she/he has attained a realistic level.

Keep in mind - the goal is not to eradicate the experience and the symptom that emerged from it - it is to integrate the experience with the concomitant learning which potentially results from any and all profound encounters. In other words - the symptom - as well as its irrational and adrenalized components - are transmuted into reality based information - and integrated as learned material.

I also agree that the exploration of earlier history and trauma experiences - especially for someone more likely to be exposed throughout her lifetime to direct and vicarious traumatization - is crucial and necessary. To not look at a trauma victim's personal pre-morbid self is to assume that all individuals encounter jarring situations with the same pre-existing constitutional and experiential templates.

How often have we found that unless we guided a client to reprocess earlier traumas, the subsequent ones did no remit - despite our most skillful and creative EMDR approaches?

Occupational trauma: treating railroad engineers with EMDR
Internationally, railroad engineers suffer from extremely high percentages of occupational PTSD. Do you know what is responsible for this phenomenon? The high frequency of suicides in front of trains, collisions with pedestrians (children, careless, inebriated or psychotic individuals) in addition to collisions with motor vehicles. When a suicidee chooses a locomotive as their death instrument - they tend to either jump in front of the train of step out onto the tracks, kneel down and make eye contact with the engineer. This becomes the engineer's lasting image, as well as the sound and odors of the impact. Additionally, pedestrians and motor vehicles often try to run a closed crossing gate - at times with disastrous consequences. It is a possibility engineers risk every time they take out their trains. Some have endured as many as five or six traumatizing incidents. Accordingly, they are a population that suffers with high percentages of acute and chronic PTSD. These engineers are the forgotten victims whose emotional, physical and family lives are often impaired if not ruined. However, it is a tragedy with a remedy - I've treated over sixty engineers on the LIRR with EMDR leading to a full resolution of all symptoms - usually in one to three extended sessions.

How soon after a traumatic event should you use EMDR?

Question: Do you think there is a problem with doing a mini-focused version of EMDR for a victim on the day of a horrific accident? I had a whole family in who were in desperate need and I wondered what the official EMDR word was. I know that recent trauma has not been consolidated and that many more fragments need to be checked. However, when you're treating a child who says he can't close his eyes without flashbacks - it's very tempting to give EMDR a shot!

Answer: It should be tempting - it is our responsibility to help those suffering any way we can. One of the misconceptions in the

EMDR world is that you have to delay treatment if it is too soon after a traumatic event. It certainly takes time to consolidate the experience - and each person does so differently. It would be cruel to deprive this boy of any relief possible. His mental tape of this traumatic imagery may proceed naturally forward or you may have to target it a frame at a time until it flows more on its own. Once the experience appears to be more consolidated - check for unprocessed pieces - particularly sounds, smells and tactile memories. Then guide the client through experience - first forward - then backward. Start with slow eye movements - up and down are most soothing until he/she is ready to close their eyes - then consider moving to bilateral sound.

The following is a process of a single three-hour session with a railroad engineer of an incident two days prior as well as three previous accidents.

This case material will examine the EMDR treatment, in one extended session, of a railroad engineer suffering from both chronic and acute P.T.S.D. as a result of involvement in four fatal incidents (all suicides in front of his train) and witnessing another suicide. Additionally, in 1991 his train collided with a tractor-trailer stalled on the tracks carrying a 100 ton piece of hydraulic equipment. The first incident occurred in 1983. This session was held two days after the most recent incident. The session spanned three hours - including extensive history taking, the EMDR treatment and debriefing.

T (Therapist): Tell me about what happened of Friday.
E (Engineer): While leaving the Kings Park Station at 4:50 a.m., one mile west of the Sagtikos Parkway, I spotted a young man sitting on the third rail. I immediately blew the horn and applied the emergency brake. He didn't react in the slightest. I turned away, as is characteristic of engineers, so as not to see the impact. I heard no noise on impact as I was driving a long nose diesel engine. The train finally stopped and the conductor called inquiring if anything was wrong. I indicated there was and he came and called the dispatcher. The conductor and brakeman walked back and saw that the body had been knocked to the side.

Two NYC cops were on the train; they went back to check and spoke to the dispatcher who asked "do you need an ambulance?" and they replied "negative" (the victim was dead). I sat and waited for three hours with a train full of passengers, which made me very uncomfortable, waiting for the Suffolk Country and railroad police to arrive. Finally a supervisor got there at 7 a.m. I got down from the train and he asked many questions and took notes. Initially they asked me to continue driving the train on its run but I replied, "I don't particularly care to take it." I didn't feel competent. I walked to the bridge over the highway and saw the crime scene. People were taking photos of the body and then they lifted it and turned it over.

T: How did you feel at that moment?

E: I felt anger at the victim (pause). Then the patrolman came and took me down to the parkway to a police car. Although it was a steep grade I was more concerned about the safety of the policeman. We sat in the car waiting for homicide and the morgue people showed up. They came, wrapped up the body and took it away. The officer then took me to Kings Park station where I waited a half an hour for the train. Because of the accident, service was still halted so I took the bus to Port Jefferson and went home.

T: What was it like for you when you arrived home?

E: My wife was happy to see me but when I told her what happened she was upset. Then I felt uncomfortable. I mowed the lawn and was running around all day Friday. I went to my daughter's, changed a flat tire and replaced the battery in her car.

T: How was it when you went to sleep?

E: I had no trouble falling asleep. I was exhausted from all of the running around. I woke up with a severe cramp in my left leg with a flashback of the approaching body. I couldn't stop thinking if somehow I could have done something sooner. (E reflected on an incident in 1998) I wish these people could see what they look like after they've been hit. Maybe they'd think twice before throwing themselves in front of a train. I was coming east out of Huntington and I approached a person standing next to the tracks. He looked towards the train, made eye contact with me, and stepped out onto the tracks. I threw the emergency brake and blew the horn. I heard the impact and saw pieces of bone, and flesh flying by. When we stopped, the front of the engine was covered with blood and a reddish brown knit hat (the victim's) was stuck to the front of the grill. I couldn't believe that after all that the hat would be sticking on the front. I felt sorry for the guys who were going to have to clean the front of the engine.

The worst incident was in 1988 in Huntington. I hit a tractor-trailer carrying a hydraulic excavator weighing about 100 tons. There was a hump in the crossing and the trailer got wedged there on the tracks. To make things worse I had a narrow field of view from about 1500 feet away from the crossing. I saw two men walking to the center of the crossing and it was then that I saw the trailer was stuck on the tracks. It was evening time to make things worse. I had the realization of what was just about to occur so I turned, crouched and grabbed a railing to brace myself. Then came the impact with a horrendous bang. Smoke filled the cab and I saw to my right the flash of a spark that immediately turned into a flame. A piece of the third rail pierced the fuel tank under the engine - came up through the floor and rammed into the engine block - which is what caused the fire. The thought flashed through my head in a split second that I was going to get burned alive. The train continued forward for a couple of hundred feet. It seemed like forever, as if a few seconds were frozen in time for hours. I heard a groaning followed by at hump as the front wheels tore off the engine. I heard things bouncing off the engine. Just when I thought the train was going to stop, the windows started to move up with an awful grinding noise, the train veered a full 180 degrees and then turned over on its side. I was trapped inside, could barely breathe and was terrified I would be burned alive. When I went to kick out one of the windows I looked down and discovered I didn't have any shoes on my feet. The impact blew them off. It seemed like forever until some guy broke one of the windows and pulled me out. When I emerged I was totally black. People were running and then the police and fireman arrived. They put me in an emergency vehicle and took me to the hospital. To make things worse my wife saw the whole thing on TV - and knew it was my train. She thought I was dead for sure until she got a call from the railroad police. Three days after the accident I started getting headaches which have continued up until this very day. The neurologist told me it would start going away in a couple of weeks and then he said months but now he tells me he

thinks it's my nerves.
T: Tell me about your headaches.
E: I get them right in the middle of my forehead. Sometimes they are milder, sometimes they're stronger. It gets very uncomfortable. I suffer from them almost every day. Sometimes two to three times a in a given day. I go through that accident spot three to four times a day. Each and every time I get a flashback. In fact every time I pass any accident spot I run a flashback. Every detail comes back to me in an instant - another incident was a Kings Park. Problems seem to happen often there. There is a crossing near the end of the station followed by a traffic light that looks like the place in Chicago where they had that nasty school bus accident. There have been five or six fatalities there in the last year or so. Well, a guy about twenty years old got out of my train which was facing eastbound at the time. He walked across the tracks without turning to look right as the westbound was coming in. When I realized he was going to be struck I turned my glance away. When I looked back I saw him tumbling and landing square in the tracks right in front of me. I can see that picture now like it just happened a moment ago.

I was called as a witness to an EBT (hearing) in Manhattan. Coincidentally, I ran into his mother and father outside the courtroom. I didn't know who they were but somehow the father glared at me with hatred. At first I was mad but when I found out who they were I felt sympathetic. At the hearing I sat directly across a table facing the victim's mother while those damn lawyers made me review each and every detail of the accident over and over for three hours straight. Looking at her face throughout was a nightmare I can't forget. The whole time I was sitting there during the procedure I had this sharp pain in my body like an arrow was sticking in my back and coming out of my chest.

E also reported - in great detail - three more accidents that took place in the 1980's.

The following is the process of the EMDR treatment held on Sunday, two days after the most recent accident:

T: What image represents the worst aspect of the incident?
E: (Image) Seeing him sit there on the third rail not responding to the horn or the sound of my train.
T: What negative, distorted belief about yourself goes with this image?
E: (Negative cognition) When you bring up the image, what would you like to believe about yourself?
E: That I did everything I could.
T: On a scale of one to seven with one being totally false and seven being completely true, how true does the statement, "I did the best I could," feel to you now?
E: Two
T: What feelings come to you now when you see that image and think of that negative belief, I am responsible?
E: (affect) Guilt - sadness.
T: What level of distress do those feelings give you with ten being the worst and zero being neutral?
E: 10 plus
T: Where do you feel that 10 plus in your body now?
E: (Body sensation) Right here in my chest.
T: (Using a Bio*Lateral* CD with headphones) I want you to hold the image together with the belief, "I am responsible," and your emotions and the sensation in your chest and simply observe where you go from there.
E: (set of 60 seconds) I kept thinking of the accident.
T: Go with that.
E: (set of 60 seconds) I thought of my dog lying on the floor peeking at me with one eye.
T: Go with that
E: (set of 60 seconds) I thought of walking to the beach in the morning with my dog like I usually do with her.
T: Go with that.
E: (set of 60 seconds) I'm still walking the dog along the beach.
T: (wondering what level of desensitization he has achieved) If you bring up the image you started with, what does it look and feel like now?
E: I just see it. It doesn't feel like anything.
T: If you put the image together with the belief, "I am responsible," what level of distress do you get now?

E: Five.
T: Go with what makes it a five for you.
E: (set of 60 seconds) My son just came home from out of town and I thought of the wedding we had last week and what a good time we had.
T: Go with that.
E: (set of 60 seconds) My relatives were at the wedding who I hadn't seen for a long time. I was thinking of how we all enjoyed being together.
T: Go with that.
E: (set of 60 seconds) I was thinking of when we went to see the stock cars. We were in Daytona and saw them practicing for the 500.
T: Go with that.
E: (set of 90 seconds) Again I was thinking of the races. I haven't seen one in a couple of weeks. The Winston Cup is on TV today and I'm looking forward to watching it.
T: Go with that.
E: (set of 120 seconds) I collect die cast cars and trucks. I found this place in Islip that sells them. I was thinking of stopping in there on the way back.
T: If you bring up the image, what does it look and feel like to you now?
E: It seems a little faded without any feelings. It looks like a distant image.
T: If you put that image together with the belief, "I am responsible," what level of distress do you get now?
E: Zero.
T: Go with that.
E: (set of 60 seconds) I'm thinking of a Chrysler with wooden sides. A '46 convertible where the wooden sides really stood out.
T: If you put that image together with the belief, "I am responsible," what level of distress do you get now?
E: There's nothing left. The picture is gone.
T: Does the positive belief, "I did everything I could," still seem like the best positive belief for you to work with now?
E: Yes.
T: If you put together what's left of the image with the belief, "I did everything I could," how true does it feel to you now on a

scale of one to seven with one being totally false and seven being completely true?
E: Six
T: Why not a seven?
E: I feel a tiny bit unsure.
T: Go with that.
E: (set of 60 seconds) I went over the whole incident from beginning to end and I couldn't find anything that I did that was wrong.
T: How true does, "I did everything I could," feel to you now on a scale of one to seven?
E: Seven. No doubt about it - the image is gone. The incident is in the past and I have no anxiety over it.
T: (installing again to deepen E's hold on the PC) Go with that.
E: Same thing.
(In 35 minutes the trauma from two days earlier was processed through completely. E then decided – with my consultation – to work with the incident when his engine collided with the tractor-trailer.)
T: What image represents the worst aspect of the incident to you now?
E: (Image) The image and sound of the impact, the smoke and the flames.
T: What negative, distorted belief about yourself goes with this image now?
E: (Negative cognition) "I could have reacted sooner and 'cause I didn't now I'm going to die."
T: When you bring up the image, what would you like to believe about yourself, now?
E: "I did the best I could and I'm safe now."
T: On a scale of one to seven with one being totally false and seven being completely true, how true does the statement, "I did the best I could and I'm safe now," feel to you now?
E: Three
T: What feelings come to you now when you bring up that image and think of the belief, "I could have reacted sooner and 'cause I didn't now I'm going to die?"
E: (affect) Terror.
T: What level of distress do those feelings give you with ten being

the worst and zero being neutral?
E: 10
T: Where do you feel that 10 in your body now?
E: In my stomach (rumbling is audible).
T: I want you to hold the image together with the belief, "I could have reacted sooner and 'cause I didn't now I'm going to die," and your emotions and the sensation in your stomach and simply see where you go from there.
E: (set of 120 seconds) I see and hear the image and sound of the impact and the smoke and the flames. I'm backing away from it and there's nowhere to go. The train slows and finally stops. I wanted to kick out a window to let the smoke out but I looked down and I saw I had no shoes on. I couldn't get to the door above or open a window. Finally someone outside opens a window and I climb out.
T: Go with that.
E: (set of 180 seconds) I pretty much relived the next part of the scene. People were running over to help.
T: Go with that.
E: (set of 120 seconds) A couple of years later I had to go to an EBT. There were 18 lawyers and 13 questioned me for three straight days. I would have preferred another accident to that.
T: Go where that takes you.
E: I know where that takes me. I hate lawyers! (set of 120 seconds) I'm glad that whole thing is behind me – the legal proceedings.
T: Can you also feel that the emotional trauma is behind you now?
E: I think so.
T: Go with that.
E: (set of 120 seconds) It's pretty much gone – I was thinking about my son. I got a die-cast racing car for him. He's into racing cars.
T: If you bring up the image and sound of the impact and the smoke and flames, what do you get from it now?
E: Nothing. The image and sound are gone. I try to see them and I can't. It's strange because I used to see and hear them many times every day – especially in my dreams. It's over. It's in the past.
T: If you put that together with the belief, "I could have reacted sooner and 'cause I didn't now I'm going to die," what level of distress do you get from that now?

E: 0
E: (set of 120 seconds) It's vague and in the past. It's not distressing anymore.
T: Go with that.
E: I'm not getting anything.
T: On a scale of one to seven with one being totally false and seven being completely true, how true does the statement, "I did the best I could and I'm safe now," feel to you now?
E: 7
T: Go with that.
E: (set of 60 seconds) It's over. I can feel safe now.
T: Go with that.
E: (set of 60 seconds) Same thing.

Processing this protocol, the most distressing of all the incidents by the client's initial assessment, was accomplished in fifteen minutes. We processed all the remaining trauma situations, each one requiring no more than five minutes to attain a full desensitization and reprocessing. As the session drew to a close I asked E what he thought of the experience to which he replied, "Good. I can't remember when I have felt this much at peace. Now I can go on with my life. Thank you." I saw E the following week and he reported no evidence of distress from any of his multiple traumas. He had one mild headache earlier in the week with no subsequent incidences of head pain since that time. In follow-up over the next three years, no reoccurrence of symptoms has been reported.

What are some advanced EMDR interweaves for treating complex cases?

It is often necessary to expand the practice of EMDR with complex patients who respond less successfully to the traditional EMDR treatment. They may present with character pathology, dissociative manifestations or other apparently intractable long-term symptomology. They may also present as non-responders who respond minimally or have adverse responses to the EMDR process. EMDR theory and practice can be integrated with the clinical principles of developmental psychotherapy. This integration – coupled with innovative treatment techniques –

enables EMDR practitioners to address comprehensively the developmental lesions that are the foundational causative factors in these clients. Human development and its vicissitudes can be conceptualized as a series of small "t" traumas, with dissociation, as a developmental organizer, as its sequelae.

What are some ways to foster EMDR's effectiveness with low responders and non-responders?

Divergent opinions exist regarding who is and who is not treatable with EMDR. Whereas treatment of acute trauma tends to yield rapid, dramatic resolution, a significant percentage of clients present with more complex situations. It is accordingly not unusual to encounter individuals whose histories, symptom and behaviors result in their presenting in session as non-responders to the traditional EMDR protocols and procedures. It is my contention that most people can be helped with EMDR. This may entail longer term EMDR, employing special attention to the subtleties of forming a treatment alliance, modification and integration of techniques and an ability and willingness to innovate a case-specific EMDR approach. Special attention needs to be given to lines of personality development, particularly regarding the ubiquitous phenomenon of dissociation. Dissociation can be conceptualized as a spectrum running from primitive fracturing on one end to the normal existence of discrete internal selves on the other. The technical approach of working with dissociative processes is describe as the locating, calling out and mapping of the separate selves or internalized objects as well as internal conflict resolution via the promotion of cooperative and integrative interaction among the selves. The diagnostic practice of developmental blueprinting is characterized by identifying both lesions (or blockages) and areas of health on the developmental lines of separation/individuation, defense mechanisms, anxiety level and super-ego functioning.

Additionally, the use of auditory and tactile bilateral stimulation presents some advantages over eye movements. Some examples are: processing with eyes closed, extended sets, having educated clients determining when to end sets, maintaining left/right stimulation in between sets and in between session use of audiotapes and CDs for symptom control, relaxation and insomnia.

PART TWO - EGO STATES

What is EMDR Ego States or Separate Selves Work?

This answer addresses an integration of EMDR with concepts that have existed in other clinical fields of thought. It is innovative primarily in the synthesizing aspect of it. The EMDR treatment approach can be used to build up strength and stability in our clients as well as reducing their painful and disabling inner conflicts. It is often assumed that the concept of separate selves pertains primarily to the defensive personally fracturing found in clients with dissociative identity disorder. However, dissociation can be conceptualized as a developmental and adaptive process found in all people. This can be illustrated by referring to the instances where you say to ourselves, "why did you do that?" or "how could you be so stupid?" These words emanate from the mildly dissociated voice of the critical self that everyone possesses. Drawing from the theory base of object relations (Edith Jacobson, et. al.) all people unconsciously internalize representations of the significant people in our early developmental years which come to exist as introjects or part objects within ourselves. We, additionally form self-representations from early in life. The interplay between these introjects is generally referred to as "object relations". In time, more mature objects develop as the archaic ones tend to remain frozen in time. By adulthood, a panoply of internalized objects exists, which I will hereto for refer to as separate selves.

The dynamic model holds that most of what human beings experience is internal and as a result of the conflicts, alliances and resolutions of these separate selves. Accordingly, our belief that how we feel is based on the events in our lives is self-deception (necessary to a certain extent). Shakespeare was diagnostically correct when he wrote, "The fault is not in our stars but in ourselves." That is not an issue of blame but simply an accurate assessment of our true locus of emotional control. As adults, the outside world, the events we face and the people we encounter serve more as triggers of our internal experience than casual factors. The concept of transference is basically the projection of an inner self on to another or as induced in treatment, on to the therapist. Working directly with these inner selves precludes the need for the use of transference to draw out, somewhat inexactly, these selves. While receiving the bilateral stimulation of EMDR, the elucidation and manipulation (in a constructive manner) of the inner selves can be greatly facilitated. You can observe how ego states metamorphosize and integrate through the basic protocol processing. However, with our most difficult - slow moving, prone to blocking clients - more direct access to the inner selves is needed.

How does one get access to different Ego States?

The following describes a technique (derived from many different concepts and orientations) for eliciting and working with the ego states - especially with the vulnerable client (VC). You first determine the level of dissociation by administering a DES, or an equivalent scale. It is key to understand, address and support with the client that the loss of contact with aspects of the self (dissociative defenses) reflects a self-protective reaction which is positive in aim. Address how these were the best modes of self-protection available to the client in their immature state - as they faced situations and feelings overwhelming to them. You then explain how as adults we can develop more effective ways to protect ourselves - methods that don't have to rob us of our contact with our emotional selves.

The following technique is referred to as "calling out the selves." Explain to your client that all people have different sides that we can refer to as separate selves. Educate and reassure - if necessary - that this does not mean you think they have multiple personalities. To illustrate, ask the client if she/he ever hears herself say, "why did you do that?" or "how could you be so stupid?" Use this as an illustration of the voice of the critical or shaming self. (Parenthetically, the negative cognition is simply the voice of these negative selves). The technique then entails setting up mental imagery that fosters the emergence of these selves. Ask whether the client would like to designate the image of standing in front of a clearing in a forest, in a safe room with a number of doors [business people often choose a board room] or an empty theatre. This approach can either be applied projectively, with some direction or a combination of the two. In the former, the client is instructed to listen for rustling in the woods or footsteps outside the office with the suggestion that it is one of her selves. As her to call in the self and let you know when she has appeared.

What do you do next?

Encourage the client to and observe (define) this self. How old is she? What does she look like? What is she wearing? What is the look on her face and her posture? What is her name? This procedure is then followed by calling out other selves. The more directive approach is to instruct the client to call out her self-critical or self-attacking self. This step is then followed by calling out her victim or attacked self. Child selves, self-doubting selves, angry or frightened selves, competent adult selves, parental selves, healer selves, etc. are often fruitful images to access. The selves can then be directed to interact in a directive or non-directive fashion aimed at communication, negotiation, leading to mutual cooperation and healing.

How do you deal with the self-aggressive selves?

I recommend using the caveat that each self is equally valuable (just like one's arm or leg) as part of the valued overall self - and the goal is not to expel or surgically remove even an abusive self. This may lead to a verbal give and take reciprocal negotiation between the attacking and attacked selves where each one states what they need - and what they are willing to offer to the other - on response to having these needs met. If a mediator is necessary, use one of the other selves or call in a mediator self. Often times the attacker will end up using their power to protect the victim self if she agrees to stand up for herself more. The victim self often provides he sensitivity or empathy the attacker self craves. In this case of this stuck client, one can call out the selves that are blocking the processing and ask them why they need to do this. Negotiate and work with healing them and possibly the processing can often continue on.

How do you reintegrate the selves before ending the session?

Closing ego state work is accomplished by guiding the client to integrative imagery with the selves. This can be aided by suggestions of the part-selves holding hands and saying her/his favorite prayer, poem, healing meditation or through facilitating the client's to accessing their own reintegration imagery through EMDR processing. When they are ready, the selves can be encouraged to slowly blend into each other. When the resulting shifts of this exercise are woven back into the EMDR protocol - substantial movement in the image and a significantly lowered SUDS rating are often revealed. This technique fosters mutual creativity and experimentation for client and therapist and can be profoundly effective with even the most stuck and difficult clients. Humans seem to be naturally able to work with this form of mental imagery especially when enhanced by EMDR stimulation. The approach also lends itself to tactile and auditory stimulation as sets can be longer and the clients have the option of closing their eyes.

Competent Inner Self Building (CISB)

Competent Inner Self Building (CISB) is a method derived from Ego State work. It is used in preparatory and ongoing EMDR treatment with the vulnerable client (VC) - those who are potentially dissociative, abreactive, and regressive (DDNOS, Attachment Disorders, BPD, etc.). It dovetails with Developmental Blueprinting (DB) with Ego States Work (ESW). Developmental Blueprinting is a concept adapted for synthesis with EMDR and presented by this author at the 1995 International Conference (tapes are still available) and was further expanded and presented by Carol Forgash and Uri Bergmann at the 1998 EMDRIA International Conference (a good listen on tape).

What is "Developmental Blueprinting?"

"Developmental blueprinting" is an ego psychological diagnostic approach that guides treatment targeted on areas of client weakness and strength. It is derived from the theories the major Ego Psychologists (Hartmann, Kris, Jacobson, Mahler et al) synthesized by Gertrude and Rubin Blanck as outlined in their book, 'Ego Psychology' (in the mid-1970's by Blanck and Blanck). The primary source for their writings was Anna Freud's landmark work, 'The Ego and the Mechanisms of Defence'. The first Ego Psychologist of course was Sigmund Freud as he developed the "Structural Model" of the mind: id, ego and superego to supersede the "Topographical Model" of the unconscious, preconscious and conscious minds.

Ego Psychology is a model of normal personality development, not of pathology. Symptoms ensue when growth is blocked by developmental lesions. This is a trauma-based model that can be used to diagnostically identify the nodal neurological points activated by the targeted EMDR protocol. Healing or reprocessing these lesions or impediments to development facilitates the resumption or normal growth. Ego Psychology also postulates that the formation of personality proceeds along a series of developmental lines from the primitive (neonatal autism) to the mature (adult health).

Some of these lines are (please note that this is not a complete list of the developmental lines):

1. Level of anxiety - from primitive fear of annihilation to signal anxiety where danger is indicated appropriately - analogous to the neocortex sorting out the limbic distress signals.

2. Separation/individuation - encompassing the stages from merger to firm self/object differentiation.

3. Superego development - no sense of right or wrong and primitive harshness (oftentimes expressed in bitterly self-critical negative cognitions) to a guiding ego ideal (the source of the positive cognition).

4. Drive taming - synthesis of primitive aggressive and sexual drives into higher functioning sublimination.

5. Perception - from having all assessments of the outside environment based on projections of self-beliefs to the accurate assessment of motivations of others - true cause and effect.

6. Identity - from a vague sense of oneself to a clear accurate experience of self and personal abilities and limitations.

7. Defense mechanisms - from the primitive denial, dissociation, splitting and projection to higher order rationalization and sublimation.

I work with the concept (see Ego States, Watkins & Watkins, Gestalt, Ericksonian, etc, etc.) of the developmental line of dissociation from fully fractured selves to normal distinct inner states of separations in self (adapted to EMDR with Uri Bergmann Carol Forgash). This is the basis of the synthesis of EMDR Accelerated Information Processing and the Ego States approach of "calling out the selves". The purpose in conceptualizing developmental lines is to recognize and identify that psychological development proceeds unevenly from line to line. A person with a primitive anxiety level may be more highly developed in the areas of superego and drive taming. These conceptualizations help us to understand (diagnose) in a thoughtful organized way and to accordingly identify areas of higher development or strengths and areas of lower development or weaknesses. This was reconceptualized in the 1970's as the range from psychotic to borderline to normal/neurotic that has led to the trauma/dissociation model.

EMDR developmental blueprinting uses these concepts to identify with greater accuracy the target zones - the areas of greater and at times profound developmental primitivity. Those of us who are conversant in these concepts have observed with amazement the rapidity in which developmental lesions are healed and movement up the development lines has been attained (i.e., separation/individuation, "it's not my fault, it's his"). Areas of strength can be targeted for further deepening by the EMDR positive installation. Healthy beliefs, self-perceptions, experiences, defense mechanisms (which I like to conceptualize as self-protection) and somatic states all can be reinforced by further processing.

Contrary to what many believe - those diagnosed with borderline personalities - as a category - are often high responders to EMDR. It is unfortunate when therapists hesitate to use EMDR with those placed in this category - as their developmental areas of weakness usually respond well to accelerated information processing. You must - of course - make as separation between those with borderline tendencies and those clearly manifesting DID - who require more intensive and careful treatment management.

What do you do if the client cannot access an inner competent self to support other ego states?

The preparatory EMDR treatment technique of Competent Inner Self-Building (CISB) can structure an adult ego state from within the client (in contrast to the more externally oriented technique of Resource Installation). Guide your client to imagine situations where she has protected (physically, verbally and emotionally) herself in an adult manner. Install the image, affect and body experience with very slow, brief sets of EM, if the client is stable enough at this time for the gentlest application of EMDR. If an inner positive self-representation begins to emerge, have her imagine being able to discuss affect laden material, being in reasonably in touch with herself with a PC like "I can protect myself better now" and install.

Another approach is to guide the client to visualize, while undergoing short sets of slow sweeps, her child self who faced feelings and situations that overwhelmed her emotionally. Ask her how her parents handled her emotions. Once she has created this image, ask her how old the child is, what she is wearing, what the look on her face and body posture is, etc.

This is followed by the core of CISB work. Ask the client to bring up the image of her competent, adult (perhaps maternal) self. If this does not occur naturally, the competent, protective, self-soothing image will have to be constructed. Gently guide the client to think of situations where she functions in a competent adult fashion (i.e., work, handling financial matters, childcare, housework or food preparation). These images can be installed as reality templates. Help the client to internalize the first image of her as a competent adult with slow sweep, short set EMs. When this is accomplished, follow with the installation of the second image and then the third. Then instruct your client to hold these three images side by side - as a three-paned triptych (it can be two). With slow Ems - these images usually blend into one with a reality derived competent adult self-created. Further install the image and its experience (cognitive, affectual and somatic) to further strengthen it. The client now has a more coherent competent self to bring to the child self in imagery (while doing slow eye movements, auditory or tactile stimulation) and to have the adult address the emotional needs of the child. Give special attention to the emotionally protective and soothing aspect of the parental interaction (which is building the internal capacities for self-soothing and self-protection). It is crucial to remember that the angry, aggressive, self attacking, shaming selves (which can be traced as the source or voice of the negative cognition) have to be called out and addressed, often times first, as they can block or undermine the effective, integrated processing. This self is usually suffering, wounded, feeling impotent and not listened to, and so is in need of healing from the competent self. This can help to detoxify it and make constructively available its energy, perseverance and goal pursuing in an ego syntonic manner.

EMDR is always an experimental process - you never know the outcome until you try out the approach. Clinical expertise and creativity allows us to observe the process and outcome and assess how to focus and strengthen it. Your client possesses inherent self-wisdom and can act as your consultant and ultimately your guide in this process.

Process recording of session using Ego States work and constant Bio*Lateral* stimulation:

The first fifteen minutes of this session entailed choosing the target and setting up the protocol with the client (C), who is a twenty-nine year old acting student. This session addressed issues that affect him in his personal life as well as inhibiting his acting. C reported losing emotional contact with himself while on stage.

During the session I employed the technical innovation of parallel protocols - selecting a recent target which leads to identifying a parallel childhood target. Starting with the recent one - a protocol is designated - leading to the same process with the early memory (oftentimes sharing the same or linked negative cognitions). C chose the recent image of himself on stage, losing emotional contact with himself with the negative cognition, "I'm never going to get it - I can't do it." His positive cognition was "I am a rich human being with a VOC rating of 2. He is an acting student so he certainly isn't a monetarily rich human being. (That's supposed to be funny). C's emotion was frustration - fear with a SUDS rating of 4 or 5. His body sensation was located in the front of his stomach.

After setting up the present day protocol I said to him, "I want you to float back to an earlier time in your life that this reminds you of" (setting up a parallel protocol).

I suspected that targeting the current issue without addressing the underpinning one might yield little sustained movement. The earlier target that C chose pertained to his mother openly having an affair while his family lived in New Zealand. Within a year she divorced his father and went to live in Australia with her lover where C saw her twice a year. His father soon remarried and daily fights ensued with C playing the role of peacemaker between his father and step-mother. Accordingly, at age seven C became a parentified child.

The earlier target image is of C being alone in a big house. The negative cognition is "There is something lacking in me." I asked him, "Does this belief connect with the other negative belief? - "I'm never going to get it - I can't do it" and he emphatically answered "yes." He chose as positive cognition, "It's okay to be by yourself." I again asked him if that went along with "I'm a rich human being" and he thought about it and again answered "yes". He rated the VOC for, "It's ok to be by yourself" at 4. The SUDS was rated at 4 and he reported feeling it in his arms. We started with the recent protocol.

T: Denotes therapist
C: Denotes client

T: Start with the image of yourself in the house with the belief, "There is something lacking in me", the emotions and the body sensations that come up with that, then put on the headphones with the Bio*Lateral* sound, and then follow your mind wherever it goes. Your thoughts may jump around, different things may come up that seem extraneous. Don't try to make anything happen.

Don't try to stop anything from happening - just go wherever it goes and observe.
C: OK
T: Periodically stop and let me know where you are at - or I'll step in and ask you to tell me where you are at. If you get into any intense emotion - don't stop in the middle of it - stay with it until you come out of it. Do you have any questions?
C: No.
T: Put the headphones on. With your eyes open or your eyes closed - just bring up that image along with the belief, "there is something lacking in me", the emotions that come up with it right now and where you feel it in your body now and just fro from there.
(Client processes)
T: Where did you go with that?
C: I went to almost the same place I go as a character in a scene where I feel like I have to produce - and there is nothing to produce. So the high point of these few minutes was the saying to myself, "is is ok that you're feeling frustrated, you're angry." There should be some expression of sorrow - some expression of pain. My body feels like I am holding my breath all the time.
T: Does your body feel that way right now?
C: Yeah.
T: I want you to just start now from that feeling your body and just go from there.
C: With the same image?
T: No, right now just start from that feeling in your body that you are describing. Just see wherever your mind goes from there.
(Client processes)
C: Holding my breath is a strong image and it makes me feel like the weight on my chest has been put there by someone. I feel my mind saying, "I didn't deserve it" or "why should I have to bear this weight which doesn't feel like my weight." It makes me feel like a little boy.
T: What are you the emotions that it brings to you right now?
C: I feel sorry for myself. I hear judgment in my voice.
T: What is the judgment?
C: That I am indulgent because I feel sorry for myself.
T: OK. (guiding towards ego states work) We are going to do a

little shift here. We are going to do an exercise to help you to work directly with that belief. We all have different sides to ourselves that are almost as distinct as different selves, under the umbrella of our overall self. There are some people who literally have different selves - but everybody - no matter whom - carries this as an inner experience. Just like you heard that judging voice, that was like the voice of another self, within your overall self.
(The client is wearing the headphones hearing the Bio*Lateral* CD all through this exercise.) What I want you to do is to imagine that you are in a theater. Your overall self walks into a theater and takes a seat. Just imagine that and stop when you are seated.
C: I am seated.
T: Tell me where you are seated in the empty theater?
C: Third row - a couple of seats off the aisle.
T: When you look from there you can see the stage?
C: Yeah.
T: You hear the footsteps offstage left or right. Tell me which side you hear them from.
C: Stage right.
T: You suspect that those footsteps belong to that self that just was being critical before. I want you to call him out onto the stage and as soon as you see him tell me.
C: I can see the empty stage but I can't make him walk onto the stage.
T: You called him out but he is still offstage?
C: Yeah, I guess so.
T: Ask him if it is OK if we talk to him, even from offstage.
C: I think that's OK.
T: In fact ask him if I can talk to him directly. He'll answer through you.
C: Yeah.
T: I'm talking with your right now, the self that's off stage. One thing I want to make clear to you is that in working in this way, the basic philosophy is that every part of Jacob is valuable, even the parts that may be struggling or causing difficulty for some of the other parts and the goal is no to try to get rid of any part. The goal is to find the parts that need to be understood, that need to be helped, that need to be healed. Do you understand that? If at any point you feel comfortable enough to come onto the stage just let

that happen.
C: Uh huh.
T: I am going to start by just asking you how old you are.
C: Seven.
T: Since we can't see you, just look down and see what you are wearing and then tell me.
C: Brown corduroys, red shirt.
T: What are you thinking about now?
C: I was thinking about walking onstage. Looking out to the audience.
T: There is only one person out there. That's your overall self. Do you feel ready to step out onto the stage?
C: yeah.
T: let yourself do it. Are you out there yet?
C: Yeah.
T: How does it feel to be out there?
C: It feels stupid.
T: In what way does it feel stupid?
C: (sighs) I don't know what I am going to do out here.
T: Now, you're the one who was making the critical statement before - right?
C: Yep.
T: Just tell me where that comes from in you.
C: It comes from a feeling of having to hold it together somehow.
T: OK. So it's not really coming from a place of real strength or security.
C: No.
T: Could it be said that you feel wounded, suffering, in some ways powerless, voiceless, helpless, in need of healing.
C: Yeah.
T: Keep in mind - that despite the fact that your attempts haven't been working for you - that you have a lot to offer to the other selves. You do have high standards. Is that true? Do you expect a lot?
C: Yes.
T: My sense is that you have a lot of determination and energy.
C: Yeah, I think so.
T: The more that you heal, the more you will be able to use these attributes for yourself, the other selves and your overall self. What

I want you to do is just think, right in this moment of what you are suffering with the most. Do you have a sense of what is really bothering you the most?
C: Not feeling - feeling like everything is out of control.
T: Where do you feel that in your body right now?
C: I feel it right here (points to stomach).
T: Just like your overall Jacob has the headphones on with the music and the bilateral sound - you have a pair of those headphones on, as well. Can you feel and hear it?
C: Yeah
T: I want you to just go with that sense of feeling out of control and the feeling in your stomach and just let your mind go from there and see where it takes you.
(Client processes)
T: Where are you with that now?
C: The feeling of being out of control means that I can't be a kid.
T: How does that feel to you?
C: It makes me mad. It makes me feel cheated.
T: Just keep on going with those feelings.
(Client processes)
T: Where did you go with that?
C: It made me think like - I'm going to grow up and be an asshole because I can't be a kid. It made me feel like my fear of getting hurt makes me always act grown up - act serious, mature. It makes me mad that I had to act mature. I feel like that took away a part of my artistic, nature, part of my creativity, my kid.
T: Is it OK if I call and adult self out to help you?
C: Yeah.
T: You're going to step back and wait. You'll hear more footsteps now - this is to your overall self. You have a sense that it belongs to your competent, adult, sensitive self. The one who is caring about people, particularly caring about children. Call him out - tell me when you see him.
C: I see him.
T: How old is he?
C: 30, I think.
T: What is he wearing?
C: He's wearing jeans and a white shirt.
T: What is the look on his face?

C: Understanding.
T: OK, I want to speak directly to him. Have you been listening to what has been going on onstage with the seven-year-old self where the critical voice came from?
C: Yeah.
T: Do you see him now?
C: Yeah, I see him.
T: How do you feel about what you heard from him?
C: I feel like someone should have told him it wasn't his job to grow up all of a sudden.
T: Let me point out something. That seven-year-old self is not in the past. He is here and alive right now. In that - would you be willing to help him with the things that he is struggling with, now?
C: Yes.
T: OK - good. We are going to go back to your overall self now - watching in the theater. I want you to observe these two selves interact with the idea of the adult sensitive competent self being there to help the seven year old self with his struggles - with his pain - and in helping him to be allowed to be a child. Just let it transpire - just observe.
(Client processes)
T: Tell me what just happened.
C: I saw the competent self - my competent self - try to explain - to nurture my seven-year-old self. He is very resistant, kind of angry, feels like the competent self is stupid.
T: Does the seven-year-old self have reasons to mistrust adults?
C: Yeah.
T: Does the seven-year-old self have reasons to mistrust adults?
C: Yeah.
T: Does your competent self understand that - appreciate that?
C: Yeah, he does.
T: When I stepped in, where had things gone between the two?
C: It felt like the competent self hadn't quite figured out the right way to approach the seven-year-old self. It felt like an impasse. I felt in me watching moments of the anger of the seven-year-old self and moments of the caring but frustration of the competent self.
T: I'm just going back to you Jacob. You told me that you did

rehab work - sometimes with teenagers and kids. I imagine that it was extremely challenging, especially with some of these kids.
C: Yes, very.
T: How did you finally get through to the kids that you reached? How did it happen? What did you do?
C: In the environment we had created - it was basically by continuing to show them love no matter what.
T: How did that work?
C: Eventually for many of them it worked. They stopped doing the things that were destructive to themselves - sometimes - or to others.
T: With some of these kids or most of these kids, did you wonder whether they were going to finally get it until they finally did?
C: Absolutely.
T: Did it leave you feeling helpless and confused, frustrated?
C: Yeah, I think so.
T: Everything you learned - everything you experienced - can you bring that with you and give the patience, hopefulness and the strength to hand in there - to give your seven year old self what he needs - just that love no matter what? Can you bring that to him now?
C: I can show him that I am here.
T: That you have patience?
C: Being committed to being there.
T: OK, I want you to step back and have your overall self watch the competent adult self bring this to your seven-year-old self and just see what happens.
(Client processes)
C: (laughs)
T: Tell me what happened.
C: I watched my seven-year-old self take in my competent adult self - observe his commitment and his care - and not his passivity - just his physical presence - which was not necessarily moving but just there - present and receptive, generous. My seven-year-old self looked at this guy and started teasing him, poking fun at him for being so grown up. The seven-year-old self started playing - letting the grownup be the grown up a little bit.
T: Can I talk to the seven-year-old self directly now?
C: uh huh.

T: How are you feeling right now?
C: Pretty good.
T: Are you surprised at all?
C: Yeah.
T: Is there any particular game or toy that you would like to have?
C: Yeah - a ball - a soccer ball - something like that.
T: Ask your competent adult self to get one for you.
C: He will.
T: Go back to your overall self and watch what happens.
C: I'm having a hard time seeing them with the ball.
T: Tell me what happened.
C: My whole self in the theater kept thinking about buying a ball. I couldn't really see what was happening in front of me though. I could imagine a game but it was the same as seeing them there with the ball.
T: OK. You hear offstage the sound of a bouncing ball. Which side of the stage is it coming from?
C: It's coming from stage left.
T: Bouncing that ball is another self of yours. This is a teenage self who's coming to bring that ball out to the seven-year-old self and to help the competent self in that way as well. Just call him onto the stage. Do you see him?
C: Yeah.
T: About how old is he?
C: Eighteen.
T: What is he wearing?
C: He's got like tennis shoes and - I don't know - sweatpants and a tee shirt.
T: What is the look on his face?
C: He has longer hair. He kind of has a joking look on his face.
T: Do you see the ball he is carrying?
C: Yeah.
Describe what it looks like - the colors.
C: It actually looks like a white volleyball.
T: What do you see now?
C: He is kind of dribbling it like a basketball - not very well.
T: Keep something in mind. Although he is there to bring this ball out to the seven-year-old self - the competent adult self is there for the teenage self as well - let the three of them interact -

keeping in mind that the ball is there for the seven year old self and he is the one who really needs to be allowed and encouraged to be a child. Just let it transpire from there. Just go a while and see what happens.

(Client processes)

T: Okay tell me what's happening.

C: The teenage ball bearer tossed the ball to the seven-year-old and the seven-year-old...

T: Yes?

C: He was screaming around the empty stage - this is a stage that's like a black box - so it has walls around it. He's acting just like a little demon - just screaming and yelling and having a good time - and then tossing the ball around with the eighteen-year-old. My competent self was just chillin' - just watching - then the other two put him in the middle and played kind of donkey in the middle with him - it was like a three way game for a while. I started to see intermixed with what was going on - images of myself melancholiness in my teenager and his sneer at life - sneer at sentimental things - cynicism - things that aren't a part of my competent self - but are a part of the teenager - and definitely a part of the seven-year-old. I saw images flashing from photographs of myself and things. I remember where the anger of the seven-year-old seemed to be what was on my face at the time. But, it felt like a family and that makes me sad. It felt like my competent self was Dad and I feel like that's good because a big part of me feels like my father was never a dad.

T: Is that where the sadness is coming from?

C: Yeah, I mean it comes from the whole idea that family was not what it was supposed to be - like everybody else's family. I never remember throwing my ball with my dad. He never let his child inside of him play with me.

(Client processes)

T: Where did that take you?

C: it took me to my relationship with Kelly and the idea of getting married and having children which is terrifying to me. I get to the edge and stop the process, break off the engagement.

T: From looking at it at the perspective of what you have just experienced, where does that terror come from?

C: Being afraid that I won't be any better than what I felt like I got

- that I am not prepared to be a parent.
T: Which of those selves who are out there feel that way the most?
C: That's hard, the seven-year-old? I don't know the answer to that.
T: Let me put it a little differently. The seven year old realized he had to give up his childhood - to ply the role of adult - to be a shock absorber with the things that were going on in the family - with your parents and the ultimately with your stepmother. I would imagine that in some ways - part of that fear comes from him having to be back in that position - when he still feels like he hasn't had enough of his childhood needs met.
C: Yeah, that makes sense.
T: Here we are talking about the seven-year-old self. You may have younger selves or older child selves - up to the adolescent self - who still struggle with that. One of the most important things to learn about how to handle your emotions as an adult - is that as a child you need to get the support and the nurturance from the outside - that you really can't give it to yourself as a child. As an adult the aspects of yourself - or the child aspects of yourself that didn't get it and are actively still with you - naturally look for it on the outside from others - but can never get it from anybody else. Whereas the child as an actual child you have to get it on the outside - as an adult you can only get it from the inside - first and foremost.
C: Yeah, one of the things that is relatively obvious to me is how much my need for approval is like psychotic. It's so total in my - I am conscious of it. I feel like I need it from the outside. When I was writing yesterday in preparation to come see you - to let some things come out - I realized that I look for approval from the most mundane, seemingly insignificant acts through to the most significant ones. You know - am I supposed to be an actor? Please tell me if I'm supposed to be an actor - I found myself in a restaurant second-guessing my decision to put my egg on my toast because - this is breakfast obviously- and looking for approval - the impulse was there. Always judging myself in the context of what I think somebody else is thinking of me.
T: In that moment - whom were you looking to for the approval in that "psychotic way"?
C: In the moment with the toast?

T: Yep.

C: I was looking to a friend of mine that was sitting next to me. The action was so unconscious until I noticed it - it was just a look to him - not even eye contact. I just felt myself look to see if he was doing it and realized that that was my impulse.

T: Which age self was looking for that approval from your friend?

C: Well, I hope it wasn't the competent adult! I don't know. It was the seven-year-old. It might have been a younger one.

T: Let's say it was the child self although it probably was a younger one. If the child self recognized and had some experience in looking to the competent adult self who is there for him - who wants to be there for him - do you think you could have handled it within yourself?

C: I'm not quite clear. If that seven-year-old - if I'd had that approval?

T: No, I'm talking about right now - you're in that situation and you realize it now. If that child-self realizes that there is an adult-self who is there just for that job - and wants to be there - and can do it better than anybody on the outside.

C: Uh huh.

T: Do you think that you could just naturally respond to it and resolve it from the inside or find a comfortable place with it on the inside.

C: Yeah, I think that that is possible.

T: Just imagine yourself there now - back in that situation with breakfast - and just allow that to flow. Don't go too far with it - just go a little bit and see what happens.

C: It feels like a domino effect. It's like one decision to give myself approval may well lead to another one. I can look at my day yesterday and just imagine the events - starting with the egg and the toast and going through the day - and thinking of moments where I caught myself looking for approval. Where instead of punishing myself for looking for approval from outside I could just give it to myself - it seems so simple.

T: I'm sure you've seen how some of the simplest things in life seems the least obvious or the hardest to see.

C: Absolutely. I feel like I am always aware of stuff like this in my life. Aware of seeking the approval and never knowing how to change the pattern.

T: I'm sure if you knew how you would have done it. You can see from this how the answers really are within yourself. Knowing that - and knowing how to access them - is a key part of finding your way out of this. I want to just take a few more steps in terms of what we are doing. Imagine that outside of the theater is a convertible four seater with the top down and your selves exit the stage - exit the theater - and they go to the car. It represents yourself and your life - and if you think back to the times when you have been struggling - your competent adult self has probably not been in the driver's seat - behind the wheel. It may have been your seven-year-old self, your two-year-old self, your fourteen-year-old self or eighteen-year-old self. Imagine that the competent adult self asserts himself - firmly yet sensitively - even using some humor - to take over the driver's seat - and to guide the other selves into the passenger seats.
C: Where do we get to go?
T: Before you think of where you're going, just tell me how the seating is arranged in the car.
C: The seven-year-old is in the shotgun position. The teenager is in the back with my overall self.
T: I want you to have your car drive off into a horizon of your choosing - and once the car is out of sight - stop and let me know.
C: It is hard to stay behind and watch them go.
T: Keep in mind that the horizon is inside yourself.
C: They are disappearing now.
(End of process recording)
Before the session ended, I returned the client to the targets of both parallel protocols - to both weave the Ego States work back into the protocols and to assess for change. His SUDS rating had diminished to a 2 on both and the images had shifted significantly to less threatening and more hopeful.

PART THREE - EMDR AND PSYCHODYNAMIC THEORY AND PRACTICE

How can EMDR be integrated with psychodynamic concepts and treatment?

EMDR was originally developed utilizing cognitive therapy theories and constructs and was initially practiced almost exclusively by cognitive/behavioral clinicians. Accordingly, the relevance and potential application of psychodynamic concepts to EMDR went largely unnoticed. However, Dr. Francine Shapiro formed the concept 'syncletic' (synthesized eclectic) as she recognized the analytic aspects of EMDR such as the significance or early childhood memories, the unconscious, free association, insight, catharsis, abreaction and symbolism (Shapiro, 1995). In fact, a psychodynamic therapist incorporating EMDR into their technique can't help but learn and recognize the value of many cognitive ideas and practices. The same holds true for the cognitive practitioner who can discover that the use of EMDR opens to them the shadowy world so familiar to the analyst. Accordingly EMDR lies at the confluence of tow great rivers of thought which is further evidence of its profound nature.

For the sake of clarity it is important that I define terms used as they often have multiple usages and meanings. In this section, psychodynamic and psychoanalytic or analytic are used interchangeably. It is essential to note that the word psychoanalysis not only connotes the method of treatment Freud devised, but refers to the body of knowledge he developed and redeveloped throughout his life in addition to the more modern theories of developmental (ego psychology and separation/individuation) and self psychology.

Later in his life, Freud faced the limitations of the treatment method he had developed and refined over many years. He admitted the need to, 'Alloy the pure gold of psychoanalysis,' by modifying his treatment model (Freud, 1919). Freud even wrote of imposing time limits in his 1937 monograph, Analysis Terminable and Interminable. Although EMDR is at its most effective when utilizing the complete protocol, you can experiment on occasion with modifications of technique that alloy the pure gold of the protocol.

EMDR practices can be integrated into a long-term, insight oriented modality in two ways. The first is to employ a fully developed protocol with trauma material or when the patient is stuck. The second approach is employed at moments when material emerges that is clearly EMDR responsive, such as distorted negative beliefs (I can't do anything right or my life has no value) or positive cognitions that can be installed (I'm not responsible, I am valuable). In these instances you might say, "Would you like to process this?" This becomes a coded communication the client understands for immediately utilizing the technique.

What are some parallels between EMDR and analytic therapy?

The EMDR process has much in common with eh analytic approach. It focuses deeply on the individual's intrapsychic mechanisms: affect, cognition, dream work, fantasies, repressed memories, somatization, unconscious defenses, conflict, self perceptions and early object relations. With the aid of EMDR, you can more effectively treat patients who are stuck, who change at a snail's pace or those who are unable to translate intellectual into emotional understanding. As the analytic clinician must be caring, sensitive, thoughtful and respectful, the same demands apply to the EMDR practitioner. The psychodynamic therapist untrained in EMDR can refer ongoing clients for adjunctive consultation with an EMDR clinician to address issues of post traumatic stress disorder, childhood trauma, or to expedite the client's treatment process. Individuals who have completed analysis, often clinicians, can receive EMDR to address unresolved issues, especially before considering a second analysis. People who have been analyzed are usually highly responsive to EMDR - as if their brains are prewired for effective processing.

A striking parallel between EMDR and the analytic approach is the use of free association. The client is instructed during EMDR to observe and report back, if they choose, any thoughts, feelings, bodily sensations or memories that occur during each set of eye movements. In EMDR, however, any lengthy discussions of these associations are discouraged as it interferes with ongoing processing. In analytic therapy, free association is used as a tool to plumb the deeper hidden meanings of symbolism expressed through dreams, screen memories and parapraxes (slips of the tongue, mislaying of objects, etc.). When material of this kind of surfaces in session - instead of asking the client to associate to it you encourage them to process it. This is a highly reliable and efficient method of helping the client understand the workings of their unconscious mind. I have also found that EMDR dramatically speeds up the associative process almost as it putting a tape into fast forward that can be referred to as 'accelerated associating.'

A vexing problem encountered in clinical work is that insight often leads to intellectual understanding which does not translate easily, if at all, into emotional integration. With remarkable effectiveness, EMDR often bridges the gap between the cognitive and affective spheres. This raises the following question: 'What is the ego's involvement with the EMDR process?' and 'Does EMDR bypass or activate the ego?' These queries deserve much thought and investigation. EMDR processing, despite apparently operating out of the conscious volitional control of the client, activates a variety of ego functions. A universal byproduct of EMDR is enhanced perspective, insight and self-understanding. This is consonant with the ego functions of perception of external reality, self-perception and the synthesis of external and internal reality.

There are interesting parallels between the analytic technique of interpretation and the EMDR cognitive interweave. Both are aimed at helping the client when they are unable to sustain the natural flow of the treatment process. In EMDR, the interweave is needed with clients presenting complicated pathologies who tend to loop, block or be limited by inhibiting beliefs. This strategy can also be used with any client when the processing becomes blocked. Analytic interpretation is used to facilitate the process of making the preconscious. Proper timing is essential for successful interpretation and is determined by addressing material that is close to breaking through to awareness.

What is the "Dynamic Interweave?"

This category denotes techniques that integrate EMDR with psychodynamic, developmental, ego and self-psychology theories and practices. It includes: listening, the timing of the interweave, the associative process, screen memories, parapraxes, dream work, resistance, transference, countertransference and treatment of character pathology. Dramatic acceleration and deepening of the psychodynamic treatment process can be observed with clients when flexibly utilizing EMDR in session. This is particularly the case in the treatment of conditions of trauma such as post-traumatic stress disorder and adult survivors of childhood abuse whom historically have been highly resistant to change. This especially applies to conditions of trauma where intellectual awareness is insufficient to ameliorate the individual's ubiquitous panic or alter their deeply held irrational beliefs and self-perceptions.

A cognitive interweave is used to facilitate movement when a client is stuck. The dynamic interweave can be aimed at accelerating or focusing processing which is not significantly impeded. A dynamic interweave, similar to an analytic interpretation, is properly timed when it elicits material that is about to break through to consciousness.

The dynamic interweave can be introduced in the form of Socratic questioning. When properly applied, this technique that can deepen and speed the resolution of conflict or trauma. It is ideally activated by a well timed, leading inquiry that will likely be responded to in the affirmative. The positive retort can then be immediately installed with great effectiveness. For example, an attuned reading of facial cues or body language might generate the question, "Are you angry?" The client is guided ipso facto into introspection, leading to a spontaneous reply, hopefully an emphatic 'yes'. This can be followed up by guiding the clients to ask themselves, "What is causing my anger?" In this open-minded procedure, the client's neurophysiological system may be stimulated to produce internally accurate material, as opposed to the unreliable responses elicited by external suggestion.

Is it possible to successfully treat character pathology and psychopathy with EMDR?

Yes, however the issue of the effectiveness of EMDR in the treatment of personality disorders, some of the most difficult individuals to treat from any orientation, including analytic, is controversial. Many experienced EMDR practitioners report having little success in treating individuals with rigid, ego-syntonic, maladaptive character structures. My experience has been otherwise, although one's treatment approach needs to be modified to address the special needs of this population. No treatment can proceed unless rapport has been established with sufficient trust placed in the therapist - this takes time and cannot be rushed. I have found that EMDR is far and away the most effective clinical tool in modifying character structure.

If you conceptualize psychopathy as a severe trauma and deprivation based condition, and if you view EMDR as capable of reaching preverbal experience, you can at least conceive that some movement can be accomplished. In traditional psychodynamic treatment, character pathology is seen as being ego-syntonic or comfortable to the client. The discomfort is to those around and affected by the client's behaviors. The goal of treatment is to transmute this pathological state to one which is uncomfortable (dystonic) to the client, where sufficient anxiety is generated to motivate the will to change. This is the core and the raison d'être of this treatment is impossible. If the clinician can draw on some special reserves and personal challenge, as well as being willing to hang in for a protracted, frustrating experience, possibility for change exists. This is a true challenge to your professional self and EMDR is a tool that allows us to accomplish what we couldn't dream of before.

How can it be done?

Start with a protocol targeting something that is distressing the client in the present. Stay with this one protocol, session after session, even if it takes months, until it is processed through to a SUDS of 0 and a VOC of 7. This provides the client with an "EMDR experience." They may then understand the possibility of processing earlier traumas. If targeting more profound issues, the second protocol will take even longer to resolve than the first one - however it will begin to reveal the defensive or protective nature of the character armor. The first sparks of human vulnerability and sensitivity may appear - they have to be fanned like the embers of a dying campfire. This can be accomplished by installing these flashes of humanness as positive cognitions. In addition to the long-term protocols, opportunities to process in ego and superego building must be done on a parallel basis - view this as the earliest of reparenting. Let yourself be charmed and mildly manipulated (within strict limits) to help engage the client. Repeatedly let them know that you care, without being gullible. This is long-term, highly challenging work. The two key factors are the age of the client (the younger the better) and their level of motivation - even if it starts out externally imposed. Once they sense that you see them for whom they really are, and still are willing to help them, a crucial bridge is crossed. I have had some success with this population, but only with the application of sustained, long-term EMDR work.

Uniformly this population has suffered repeated early traumas. Accurate EMDR targeting of these experiences results in the softening of the rigidity and increased internal and external relatedness. Repeating a point for emphasis, it is crucial to stay with one protocol until full desensitization and reprocessing has occurred. Significant movement on the SUDS and the VOC will often times require many weeks and at times months and accordingly many therapists erroneously believe the work is ineffective and abandon it. Of course, active use of the cognitive interweave is necessary to bridge the many gaps found with this population. Additionally, a combination and variation of different techniques is required. High counts of repetitions of bilateral stimulation can accomplish movement that briefer repetitions would not accomplish with the concretized material and deeply distorted beliefs. Also, repeated returns to target - even if processing is still occurring - seems at times to jar lose rigidly entrenched beliefs and perceptions. Active targeting of ego-syntonic pathology can initiate a slow emergence of more healthy and appropriate ego-dystonic mentation.

How does transference and countertransference emerge in EMDR?

When introducing EMDR into an ongoing analytic therapy process, many questions must be considered such as, "What is EMDR's effect on resistance and transference?" My experience has been that resistance emerges to EMDR as it does to the analytic treatment process. The greater anxiety appears to be in giving up the secondary gains of passivity and internalized aggression in the form of self-punishment. However, the making conscious of unconscious material appears to occur with less resistance, perhaps because of the concurrent desensitization and gained perspective that so often accompanies it with EMDR treatment. Transference responses to EMDR usually relate to the relative speed and ease that movement is accomplished as contrasted with the painstaking and incremental changes which come with more traditional treatment. In the short term, EMDR may alter thinking patterns, awareness and symptoms however character is not easily effected. It is fascinating to observe the conflict in clients who symptomatically no longer need treatment yet find their attachment to the therapist and the holding environment remaining undiminished. I have also observed occasional subtle transference reactions regarding the magical quality, implied power and intrusion of the therapists performing EMDR.

Obtaining EMDR training and integrating it into one's practice is not an emotionally simple venture for the analytic therapist, especially one who is institute trained. He/she can struggle with the guilt of violating allegiances or the fear of being exposed, cast in a negative light and ostracized by teachers, supervisors and colleagues. A dramatic shift away from the way one has practiced successfully and comfortably for years raises for one with EMDR training to become and "EMDR dropout" who ceases using the technique. We all have struggled in doing treatment with the ubiquity of our countertransference reaction to our clients. In employing EMDR, the analytic therapist has to consider countertransference issues such as - whether they are using it out of frustration to control or distance themselves from the client - whether they are using it too much or too little - and to face the fear of what repressed traumas may emerge.

The issue of negative transference likely appears more in the EMDR process than we tend to realize. Not only can the power of the EMDR make us appear to clients as the "good fairy" - concurrently as the "evil genius" or Dr. Caligari. Our effectiveness may be perceived by the client's primitive self as a boundary invasion. Our ability to remove symptoms and negative beliefs can feel to clients like taking away their transitional object, which they hold tightly for the familiarity of its smell and feel. This is especially so if the early maternal or paternal relationship was aggressivized by trauma or abuse and the transitional object is accordingly aggressivized.

The client can also respond to our EMDR methods by either holding in or expelling out either the process, or us, like the toilet training two-year-old, especially if he/she was traumatized during this period. Anal retention can be observed in the client who refuses to give us any information, who states "nothing is happening" or "it's not working" - thwarting our efforts to explore their responses. Anal expulsion can be viewed in the client who either talks during the processing no matter what we do or speaks incessantly and won't let us interrupt him in between sets.

Our countertransferential response can be to either force an EMDR "enema" on the retentive client or to technically "cork" the expulsive one. This reflects that we are being triggered and losing our ability to empathize with the client, their need for self protection and their traumatized state.

Some clients may transferentially experience the EMDR as an abandonment because the therapeutic relationship is different during the EMDR protocol - unconsciously perceived as if their therapist has left and been replaced by someone else. This is especially so in ongoing treatments where EMDR is introduced midstream. The locus of the holding environment provided by EMDR is more internal and less object-related in contrast to dynamically-oriented treatments. This can be ameliorated to some degree by building in regular talking sessions or times to talk more extensively during the EMDR sessions.

On the issue of technical interventions or interweaves one must be careful not to confuse - inappropriate, countertransferential intrusions into a client's processing which is moving apace - or the converse - when the therapist eschews interweaves which are needed to address the blockages to healing. The technical ideal is to accurately set up the protocol which defines and drives the target material - and step out of the way as the client's processing, interrupted only by limited verbal intercourse at the end of each set, naturally leads to full desensitization and reprocessing. Increasingly we find that this does not occur, as overriding negative self-beliefs, often the voice of the critical self, block movement and change. More distressing is when the client runs a massive dissociative wall protecting against a terror state (often emanating from profound preverbal trauma) which at times resists all our attempts at resource installation and restructuring.

A technical intervention is not taken to "make the client feel better." It is used to help the client resume or improve their processing. The more we use EMDR - the more we see how complex a process it is. We are gaining more direct access to the most complex mechanism known at present in the universe - the human brain - which contains over four quadrillion interconnections. The earlier the trauma, the more repeated and profound it is, the more it has insinuated its way into the brain and its various structures. It is a challenge to continually refine the knowledge base and practice of EMDR to make it more effective when faced with the conditions where it proceeds glacially or not at all.

Therapists carrying their own trauma histories need to be vigilant that their own experiences are not interfering with how they are responding to their clients. Since the days of Freud - it has been a requirement to those in analytic training to undergo what used to be called a "didactic" analysis - to both experience the process first hand and to work through issues that would likely become countertransferential. It bears consideration that we voluntarily undergo a significant EMDR treatment for the same reasons - as well as to foster our own healing processes. There is efficacy to a longer-term (6-18 months) exploratory EMDR treatment for this purpose. This is often necessary to reprocess our characterological issues.

What are "Part Protocols?"

There are ways of moderating EMDR so that it can be both tolerable and useful earlier in treatment with certain fragile and early-traumatized clients. This entails a redefining of our thinking and practice. If broken down into more tolerable doses, the EMDR experience can be less powerful and more tolerable. This starts by choosing current day target that is not overwhelming and utilizing parts of a protocol, such as just the image, negative cognition or affect (I would keep away from the body sensations initially as so much trauma memory tends to be stored somatically). Proceed with exceedingly slow eye movements for the initial one or two sweeps. Allow a greater than usual amount of time for talking in between these abbreviated sets. Very gradually increase any aspect of this process - as it appears the client is able to comfortably tolerate more. If a client cannot tolerate slow, gentle processing - this presents valuable diagnostic information and of course the process should be discontinued immediately. If this graduated approach is tolerable at a low level - it will often contribute to enhanced ego functioning which can gradually guide the client toward to approach full protocol processing.

Adjunctive EMDR Therapy: What are key issues to anticipate when doing EMDR with a client in treatment with a primary therapist:

1. This process must be portrayed - from the outset - to the client and to the referring therapist - as a team-effort of three - with the client as the team leader (as the work revolves around her and she is contracting for this approach).
2. Never enter into this arrangement unless you have full confidence in the professionalism and clinical acumen of the primary therapist.
3. Determine - by interviewing the primary therapist carefully - both the efficacy of this three-way approach - based on diagnostic reasons as well as where the client is at in their treatment. Be careful of a therapist who is deliberately or unconsciously trying to dump their client.

4. The therapist must agree to attend the first session and return whenever you request it. The primary therapist must take the main responsibility for the treatment and maintain regular contact with you.

5. Screen the client carefully as you are performing adjunctive work with the goal of completing it in as few sessions as possible. If you have exceeded ten sessions - your involvement is likely beyond adjunctive. The best cases are those with discrete PTSD and patients stuck on an issue - and not pressed up against a wall of terror.

6. Triangulation will occur - anticipate it - prepare for it - deal with it immediately and whenever it occurs. If handles properly it doesn't have to be a problem - it may be a clinical opportunity. But if the client wants to terminate the primary therapist and continue with you, WATCH OUT!

7. DO NOT ACCEPT MANAGED CARE OR REDUCE YOUR FEE - BUT DON'T RAISE IT EITHER. YOU ARE BEING CALLED IN FOR YOUR SPECIALIZED EXPERTISE ON A SHORT-TERM BASIS. IF YOUR STRUGGLE EXCESSIVELY WITH WHETHER YOU ARE WORTH IT, CONSIDER SEEING AN EMDR THERAPIST AND MAKING THIS ISSUE YOUR FIRST TARGET.

8. If all of these conditions are met, Adjunctive EMDR Consultation (AEC) is both clinically and financially viable. When can you be sure of this? When it is a win/win/win situation for you, the primary therapist and most of all for the client.

Q & A regarding EMDR, ADD and personality disorders:
Question:
I am requesting advice regarding a woman who was referred to me because she "failed" many other treatments and had heard of EMDR. Her immediate issue was her inability to make up her mind regarding a financial issue.

Answer: Talk about skimming the surface! What does this really mean deeper down? (A question that should be kept in the back of your mind).

Question: Her list of diagnoses includes recently diagnosed ADD, obsessive personality, generalized anxiety, and (my diagnosis) mixed personality disorder with borderline and narcissistic traits.

Answer: EMDR is a wonderful diagnostic process - as the treatment unfolds the processing will reveal the most accurate and comprehensive diagnostic picture.

Question: This client is alternatively critical and apologetic; demanding and conciliatory. She talks a great deal and finds it difficult to comply with EMDR protocol (e.g.) she won't give me a SUDS level because she can't make up her mind). She can identify plenty of potential targets (she was raised by a borderline mother and narcissistic father) and has some good insight - but is highly defended. I have tried to use resource installation with her, but she perseverates on negative thoughts and images.

Answer: The case presents a challenge to you clinical acumen, creativity, flexibility and willingness to wrap the EMDR around the client - not to force her to fit into a model she can't work with at this time. The key is to comfortably flow with her wherever and however she takes you on her journey.

Question: I have been working with her for more than 8 sessions, trying to accommodate her wherever possible while setting limits; sometimes this appears to be helping.

Answer: Please elaborate - if she is trying to intentionally manipulate you and defeat the process - active management of the treatment process is necessary. If she is doing the best she can - then structuring - as opposed to educating and working with her at the level she is at - is the way to go.

Question: She requests long, repeated EM sets and sometimes declines to give feedback, but then she will describe shifts or reports dreams between sessions. This is frustrating - quite unlike other EMDR clients I have worked with.

Answer: There is irony in your frustration with this client's not meeting your expectations and not cooperating with the text-cookbook recipe. It sounds like she is inducing a countertransferential reaction in you - letting you know how she feels or has been treated. The treatment approach - should not be determined by our comfortableness or our need to know and understand - but by following the client wherever they need to lead us.

With EMDR you can work with a lack of feedback - as long as you sense that the client is processing - not triggered into an adverse response (you usually know this when you see it) and shifts are happening during the week - especially activated dreaming. A question that would be very valuable to have your client answer is - do you feel, think or act at all differently during the week? This is our ultimate confirmation the process is having an effect.

Question: Do you think either the ADD or the personality disorder makes her an unlikely candidate for EMDR?

Answer: It would be tragic - and a classic novice faux pas - to not consider her as a potential EMDR candidate. Treating her can be like working with a combination of a terrible two child (who need tremendous support and understanding - and define themselves by saying "no!") and a labile, limits testing midadolescent torn between the need for autonomy and dependency on her parents. Don't give up the ship! I have done full protocols with kids, teens and shame-based adults who couldn't or wouldn't share info and guided them to a zero SUDS and 7 VOC without ever knowing the topic. Should your need to know supersede the client's need for control? Keep in mind that borderline manifestations are ego weakness and developmental deficits, which respond powerfully to EMDR - fostering perspective, synthesis, etc.

It sounds like the treatment is working. Flow with her and try taking a SUDS like we do with kids - by having her hold her hands apart wide for distress and bringing them together for less or none. Don't be afraid to play, share creativity and even have fun with her. Always remember - it is the challenging cases that are the best learning opportunities.

PART FOUR - BODY PROCESSING

In Francine Shapiro's development of the EMDR treatment method she highlighted the importance of the role played by the body (soma) in the processing experience. According to her empirical findings, physical sensations can be activated by attending to a traumatic memory, may be a component of the sensory experience of the target trauma itself (i.e. an accident or an attack) and are additionally elicited by the resonance of the negative cognition. Accordingly, body sensations are invaluable focal points for EMDR processing. The clear body scan is a fundamental criterion used to determine the competition of a treatment protocol.

My beliefs on body sensations and pain have been influenced by my personal experiences with somatic symptoms. I suffered from migraine headaches in my adolescence (I now get a migraine once every ten years!), intense abdominal pain in my early twenties, a remaining tendency to somatize easily as well as a history of anxiety, discrete phobias and occasional panic attacks. I have observed myself transmuting intense feelings of anxiety directly into a burning sensation in my abdomen. At another time - it started with the burning which I observed flow directly into anxiety. A key was when I asked myself what was bothering me (pre-EMDR days). When the underlying issue became conscious, the anxiety and the abdominal distress both vanished. I also realized that when I had migraines I was devoid of emotion - and self-examination led me to realize that I was experiencing sealed off rage. The "blinding" intensity of the rage was matched by the intensity of the pain of the migraine. Encountering and releasing these emotions reduced the need for their bodily expression.

In addition to self-observation, I have processed somatic sensations with thousands of clients using EMDR. I have noted the high correlation between body fluxing - ongoing moving of body sensations - and anxiety conditions - usually with a panic component. In addition I have seen the direct targeting of body sensations often leading to release of its affective content.

My approach with clients I treat with EMDR is to give special attention to where the client is at emotionally, physically, spiritually - especially in their intertwined mind/body/spiritual self. Whether the client is coming to me for help with an emotional or relational issue, a physical condition or soul searching - I never look at the mind, body or spirit in isolation - especially for people with pain syndromes and disease processes. The client is seen in the context of their organic whole, and the interplay between its different components.

How can EMDR be used diagnostically with body experience?

You can use EMDR as a diagnostic tool both for physically (especially pain syndromes) and psychologically-based conditions. The value of EMDR as a diagnostic tool, in my experience, has been to some degree overlooked. However, the cardinal rule that applies in using EMDR as an emotional treatment tool - don't presuppose anything - also applies when addressing medical and surgical patients with EMDR. As with any EMDR process, the client needs to be thoroughly educated - how it works and how it may help them. This aids the client in self-defining - and defining for us - what they truly want and need. By letting knowledgeable clients take the lead, you avoid imposing your beliefs on them. By nature, they would tend to reject external defining both mentally and physically - leading to a greater chance of treatment failure.

I have integrated a number of Dr. John Sarno's ideas and practices on TMS (Tension Myositis Syndrome) with EMDR. The question regarding body pain starts diagnostically - how much is physically-based? How much is emotionally-based? What is the ratio of the physical to emotional genesis of the pain? How much is emotional stress secondary to the physical condition exacerbating the organic pain? EMDR can help answer some of these questions via reprocessing body experience, belief, affect - targeting the causative incidents.

How can you work with body sensations in EMDR?

Traditional processing is initiated by inducing eye movements while the client simultaneously holds the image, the negative cognition, the associated affect and the awareness of body sensations. However, it has been empirically demonstrated that effective processing can be successfully elicited by simply targeting the somatic experience when the image and cognition are absent. Also, there can be value to deliberately targeting body sensations for processing in selected situations - despite the availability of images, cognitions and affective material. Additionally, use of imagery associated with body sensations ("if you imagine the sensation is caused by something in or on your body, what would it be? Is it solid, liquid or gas? What is its size, shape, color, weight, temperature, texture, etc.?") coupled with repeated returns to the body sensations can accelerate and focus processing. As the processing continues - the body sensations and imagery tend to diminish - usually towards smaller size, lighter weight and softer colors. Ideally this process continues until there is no body distress detectable. Processing can then resume or can be returned to target to observe if this interweave has appreciably changed the image and/or SUDS level.

Focused targeting of body sensations can also facilitate processing with reduced agitation for clients who tend to respond with problematic levels of flooding, regression or dissociation. There is particular efficacy using body processing in the treatment of somatically charged conditions such as hypochondriasis, panic disorders, character pathology (armor) and chronic pain (i.e. TMJ, muscle spasms, headaches, irritable bowel syndrome, asthma and chronic fatigue).

How can Bio*Lateral* CDs and tapes be used outside the office in addressing physical issues?

Bio*Lateral* Sound Recordings provide EMDR therapists the flexibility of having appropriately chosen and prepared clients benefit from bilateral stimulation outside of the office with insomnia, agitation, relaxation, pain control and managing the stress of illness and hospital stays. I have found it extremely helpful in preparation for surgery and other medical procedures. It is particularly effective in quelling and at times eliminating presurgery and preprocedure anxiety in the waiting room. Wearing the headphones during surgery and other procedures performed under local anesthesia, can also both help the client stay relaxed and in control as well as support the doctor's appropriate "patient management." This is also applicable to dental procedures and dental phobias. Use of the Bio*Lateral* technology also affords the EMDR therapist, where appropriate, to use phone EMDR for hospitalized or homebound clients unable to come into the office. This can be done in a full session format or segmented into 10 to 15 mini sessions conducted more frequently as needed.

With cancer patients EMDR can address a multiplicity of issues. These include dealing with illness and possible mortality issues, coping with pain, procedures and separation from family and home, addressing emotional connections of the illness to prior traumatic (emotional and physical) events and enhancing alternative approaches such as visualization and positive imagery.

Of course in the treatment of dysmennorhea, underlying bulimic or anorexic tendencies - an earlier history of sexual abuse should be looked for in the history taking and EMDR processing. A full medical workup has to be done with all physical conditions to rule out or rule in possible causes. When the course is organic, EMDR can be used not only to deal with the emotional overlay, but also as an augmentation of the medical treatment using body sensations and imagery.

A key aspect of my approach with body issues is the use of tactile bilateral stimulation - which goes well beyond hand tapping. The technique of alternating hand (or foot where needed or appropriate) stimulation is done by bilaterally pressing acupressure (or Reflexology) points on lines of meridians and on areas of discomfort or sensitivity. Many clients have found this to be a less agitating form of processing which fosters positive body experience - including sensations of warmth and energic flow. The application of this technique, which naturally incorporates human contact and therapeutic touch, has efficacy in the treatment of medical conditions, especially with those in pain and/or severely debilitated.

Q & A on use of Bio*Lateral* with pain:

Question: I would like to know how you are using your tapes with pain reduction. I have a gunshot victim whose arm was impacted by the bullet that went through her back and exited through her neck. The nerves in the left arm were apparently damaged producing severe pain in her hand as well as arm paralysis. The NC is that she may never regain use of her arm - which is in fact also the reality.

Answer: If I read you correctly, the NC is a reality statement - not one that is irrational or distorted. If this is true, it will not process out and needs to be changed. Pain issues are extremely complicated and depend greatly on the individual's pre-injury emotional, body and pain profile. Were there any predating injuries or traumas? Childhood development issues also play a key role in how a person responds later to injury or pain. Using the headphones straight through the session, I would target the traumatic event and any body sensations that arise from the affect before targeting the injury pain. If it is a discrete trauma, it should process through except for the existence of future disability and pain. After the protocol is completed, determine if any shift has occurred in the arm pain or finger numbness. Targeting these sensations, especially using imagery, may help to further modify the pain.

Use of Bio*Lateral* CDs and tapes outside of the office is particularly helpful when pain is evident or spikes, or when upset or agitation about the pain or event occurs. This is particularly the case if the person has difficulty with falling asleep or waking in the middle of the night.

Q & A on Somatic Issues and Ego States:

Question: One of my older clients (58) had many regrets about how she raised her children. She had problems with her bowels, although I don't really know the specific symptoms for "irritable bowel syndrome." We uncovered extreme sadness as she began to process her NC (something like "I have to pay"). There were specific events that she truly agonized over - perhaps 10 in all. Her SUDS went back up when she returned after incomplete processing the week before, but she was able to complete the SUDS processing in the next session. Her PC was something like "It's over now; I don't have to pay anymore." We plan to install that this week.

I think the most important thing in this was that she was able to take something that felt so enormous and amorphous and

give it a name and a structure. This was an exciting session for both client and therapist. What are your observations?
Answer: Your defining of the events is an excellent refinement that warrants further usage and feedback. I have found that anything that provides further definition for the individual helps activate and deepen the process. Another example is defining body sensations with imagery: "If there was something in or on you creating that sensation, what would it be? What is its shape, size, color, weight, temperature, etc?

Some clarification is necessary to properly answer your question. How were her IBS symptoms affected by the reprocessing? How much her body was/is speaking for her (crying, screaming) needs to be understood for where it was and is. Remaining somatic distress can be targeted directly or in other cases be used as a diagnostic indicator of more buried material/trauma. One needs to proceed cautiously with direct targeting of extreme body pain as flare ups, emergence of overwhelming affect (terror states) or dissociative phenomena, which can short-circuit the process, may occur.

Another question is, "What remains of your client's self-critical/attacking tendencies?" A way to both diagnostically determine as well as treat this is through using the separate/part selves/ego states/imago approach. This is subsumed under a targeted protocol as well as catalyzed by bilateral stimulation (ideally auditory or tactile so client can close their eyes and do longer sets).

Have your client imagine her overall self, standing in a clearing in a forest, or in the front row of an empty theater - then tell her to listen for footsteps in the trees or offstage. Suggest that it is her self critical or attacking self - then ask her to call her out and let you know as soon as she is visible. This usually works quickly. When the client sees her ask, "How old is she? What is she wearing?" What is the look on her face? What is her posture?" This is a defining technique analogous to the one you conceptualized.

You now have direct access to a crucial, damaging and wounded part of her. The first step is to reassure the critical self (CS) that the goal should never be to banish or destroy her. This is equivalent to challenging a client's resistance. Then help identify that this self is a wounded self who feels voiceless, unrecognized, powerless and helpless. Remind the client that we don't cut out our wounds, we try to heal them. Also point out that this CS has valuable things to offer if she can be healed, such as determination, perseverance, high standards, etc.

Healing the CS can be attempted in a variety of ways. You can work up a protocol and do EMDR with her (having her listen to the client's tones or feel the tactile stimulation). You can also identify, call out and clarify a competent adult self, loving parental self, spiritual self or healer self. If none exists - she can be created by processing in key positive experiences the client has experienced in reality - followed by coalescing them. With imagery put the caring, competent helper-self together with the wounded critical-self with the task of listening and ministering to, supporting caring and healing her. If the CS is balky, encourage the client to use her patience just as she would in approaching angry, hurting child. If the client is still feeling abdominal pain you can have the helper put her hand on the stomach of the CS to soothe it. End with a reintegration exercise where the selves hold hands in a circle, recite their favorite prayer, hymn or song and slowly blend together. Return to the original target in the protocol to see how this exercise has shifted it and to reintegrate (connect the neural networks) the subsumed imago interweave into the protocol. Then do some more processing of the protocol to further internalize the experience.

What have been your experiences in targeting pain with RSD (Reflex Sympathetic Dystrophy) patients with EMDR?

Although I have worked with body processing for many years - I have a few recent observations from my work in the pain clinic of ProHealth - a local innovative medical center. Those I have encountered there are often at the end of the line in seeking treatment options. Some of their pain is of unknown origin, some are from pernicious conditions such as RSD (Reflex Sympathetic Dystrophy). I had usually targeted the body sensations or areas of pain directly, oftentimes with remarkable results. In my work at ProHealth this approach often resulted in an exacerbation of both physical and emotional symptoms. Diagnostically this suggested to me that I was not only working with clearly dissociative conditions, but oftentimes ones of unusually early origin. I had to quickly recalibrate my treatment approach using mild trial and error approaches.

The method I know find most appropriate parallels the one I evaluate and treat patients with dissociative disorders. Taking a comprehensive history, getting a DES or other measures, and establishing a secure treatment relationship and support system is recommended for patients with unusual, extensive or unresponsive pain syndromes. When introducing EMDR, it is with a current, live issue presented as, "what is bothering you or on your mind now?" A protocol is built around this with careful observation of body sensations. I have usually observed that the body sensations arise in the usual areas patient's report (chest, stomach, neck, head) distinct from the sites of intractable pain. It is as if the permanent pain derives from another place and time, has a life of its own, and quite literally is extremely early in development.

In introducing EMDR, I begin with extremely slow eye movements, literally taking 15 to 30 seconds each sweep across, for only one or two repetitions. I then stop to check closely how the patient is processing. If any extreme abreaction or switching takes place I immediately interrupt the process. However, with this gentle approach, I find this rarely happens. Under close observation, I very gradually increase the pace and count of the eye movements. I have found with this approach, basic protocols can be processed in a way that begins the structuring or ego building process. I have also observed - surprisingly - that the body sensations elicited by the mild target will process out as usual - with little or no effect on the refractory pain symptoms. This certainly suggests a dissociative quality and shows how the body experience can be split off, just as the self can be.

Gradually these patients can tolerate deeper targets, particularly the trauma of the onset of their pain - often an accident, surgery or body trauma has elicited it - as well as their fears regarding future prognosis. Of course use of resource installation - safe, secure, serene place installation - is an essential part of the process. I have found specific targeting of separate selves, parts or ego states quite valuable. This is especially helpful in identifying and healing self critical and attacking selves as well as body representations.

Throughout this extended treatment process, close observation of any metamorphoses in the resistant areas of pain is conducted. This provides indication of any deeper changes that may be beginning as well as the patient's readiness to address deeper trauma. It is yet to be determined to what degree resolution of the preverbal traumas can shift these most resistant pain syndromes. However, with ongoing integrative, innovative development of state of the art EMDR techniques and the truest use of the bipersonal healing relationship, change remains within the realm of possibility.

How can one help treat high blood pressure with EMDR?

Start by targeting the question, "Is any stress or emotional component contributing to your BP elevation?" Process any material that emerges. Have the client to produce an image of their circulatory system as it is now and observe how it appears to be problematic. Then ask him to produce a picture of how it should look. Have the client hold both pictures side by side and suggest that the current picture slowly take on the characteristics of the ideal one. Then imagine a switch or knob that can facilitate the picture and blood pressure changing. If he resists this process, encourage your client to ask himself why and process the material that emerges.

Another approach is to imagine that the blood stream is composed of rivers and lakes. Process the image with the idea that the lakes and rivers will change geologically in a way that will cause less rush (pressure) of water.

Q & A on EMDR and Stuttering:

Question: Several weeks ago I used EMDR to help a boy who stutters reduce his fear of going into public places. The target image was of him going into a department store. The NC was "Everybody's looking at me and judging me" and the PC was the opposite. VOC was 4. SUDS was 7 with the emotions of anxiety, fear, feelings of inferiority. At the end of the session the VOC was

5 and the SUDS was a 3. When he came back the following week he reported that he'd been able to go into a store with relative ease and therefore didn't to complete the processing. This man was raised by a stern, controlling father and an overprotective mother. Now that he has asked me to help him with his stuttering I feel that I should complete the processing of the store fear memory. What would you advise?

Answer: Clients will often misperceive that they have gone far enough with a protocol when there is a shift - they feel and function better - even when they have not reached a zero SUDS. At times it is lack of information although fear of opening further material can be involved. I would suggest the educational approach first and the exploration piece (using bilateral stimulation) second. This client not only needs to process through his current anxieties, he needs to target childhood memories. You can almost imagine him overwhelmed with fear, guilt and shame while being confronted angrily for an answer and being unable to come up with the words. How this is physiologically carried in his current stuttering raises interesting questions. Only after the current and past issues are targeted and reprocessed, can the stuttering be directly targeted effectively.

Q & A on different forms of neurological stimulation:

Question: I was involved in a group discussion in which active ingredients were discussed extensively. Some claimed that there was plenty of research supporting the idea that eye movement was not necessary (but isn't plenty an exaggeration?). But subjectively some form of stimulation or processing that elicits integration of hemispheric styles would seem to have quite an impact. I think there are stimuli that can substitute for eye movement or other alternating bilateral stimulation to various degrees, but I just can't see giving it up. I'll wager that in time, there will be more evidence in favor of alternating bilateral stimulation.

Answer: With my involvement in bilateral sound and tactile stimulation I have looked into a great deal of the technology available beyond the EMDR world to assess the applicability to the processing we stimulate. I checked out Hemisync which describes using binaural sound (different designated sound frequencies played into each ear) and determined that it was not bilateral (confirmed by their sound engineer). Regardless I proceeded with a few clients to try using Hemisync with the EMDR protocol. I observed very faint processing with little change obtained with the SUDS. I was tried using the Hemisync with hand tapping which two clients seemed to find disruptive. I have also looked Andrew Weil's CD that utilizes psychoacoustics and have not observed any processing comparable to the left/right eye, sound or tactile stimulation.

I have tried using slow and up/down eye movements simultaneously with my tapes and have found some positive responses, especially with blocked processing. I believe we have just scratched the surface when it comes to understanding and making controlled use of bilateral stimulation as well as other developing techniques.

Part Five - Defining and Redefining EMDR: Performance and Creativity Enhancement

What are you ideas and experiences with EMDR Performance Enhancement?

As I come from a different clinical background than most who work in the area I refer to as Performance Enhancement (also called as Peak Performance or Sports Psychology) the diagnostic and treatment approach I employ (developmental and object relations) tends to vary from the norm. My philosophy and conceptualization of performance issues also tends to cover a wider scope than many. Accordingly, my ideas and approaches cannot be organized into or subsumed under one or two basic protocols. I will, however, attempt to present these ideas in the most succinct manner possible.

The 9 Guidelines for Performance Enhancement:

1. Performance should be seen in the larger context of life experience, meaning and self-perception and is limited when looked at primarily in terms of sensory input and response, thought (beliefs) and behavior.
2. Performance is an every day, all day issue of life for everyone including all interactions with others and within ourselves (Ed Koch used to repeatedly ask of his performance as mayor of New York City, "How'm I doin'?").
3. How we experience present day performance is influenced by the accumulation of performance experiences dating back to birth (intrauterine experience?). How our parents and caretakers respond to our early performances such as nursing, rolling over, smiling, cooing and babbling, walking, talking and toilet training - forms the foundation for our later performance experiences (both inner and outer). Parents can respond with positive mirroring (Kohut) such as excitement and reflections of, "Look what Ellen did! She rolled over!" or "Billy, what a wonderful picture!" However, if parents respond adversely or perhaps more damagingly by ignoring these early performances, negative strata

accumulate which develop a performance sense of "I am bad" (shame development) or "I am invisible" (I don't exist). Early social experiences with young friends and in going off to nursery school and kindergarten are key to our performance histories as they are usually the first structured group performance and evaluation experiences of life. EMDR processing of present day performance anxiety often yields humiliation memories from school, especially elementary school.

4. Performance and social anxiety are dynamic phenomenon which originate with negative self-beliefs and images, mostly unconscious and formed earlier in life. These inner perceptions are silently projected out into the minds (perceived thoughts) of the observers (audience or others and are then erroneously experienced as external. Through reintrojection, the performer's tendencies towards anxiety and shame are then activated further affecting both internal experience and actual performance, forming a negative loop. This may develop into a downward spiral which at its worse leads to an avoidance or cessation of the activity. Identifying how these dynamics develop and are played out for the individual can help to expose and unravel them, especially incorporating EMDR exploration and targeting of the formative experiences.

5. The projected negative self-perceptions, beliefs and self-statements (which we identify as negative cognitions) often emanate from distinct ego states or separate selves, even in non-DID individuals. These are self critical and/or attacking selves that can be identified and worked with directly. These selves are in need of healing as they usually feel voiceless, powerless, disenfranchised and are suffering. They also, when healed, have energy, assertiveness and determination that can serve the overall self. Other selves (parental or spiritual/healing) can be brought to the aggressive self for healing and/or direct protocol work with this self.

6. Secondary gains of performance blocks need to be considered and evaluated. Hidden secondary gains often play a role leading to avoidance and escape. For the child or adolescent prodigy, the question of, "who am I performing for, myself or my parent (coach/teacher)" often lurks silently. This issue continues into the adult life of the prodigy who may be unknowingly

rebelling or calling out for recognition or help. It is not uncommon for prodigies to be abused in childhood, especially in relation to the development of their giftedness. I have worked with more than one concert pianist who were either hit in the back of the head by her mother/teacher or verbally humiliated by a teacher between the ages of five and ten. Those in the public eye are treated as commodities by corporations and fans and accordingly experience being divorced from their true selves. "They don't like me for who I am, they like me for what I do." This deepens the traumatic experience of abandonment and exploitation and tend to intensify the performers need to defensively rely on narcissism and dissociation. This is a pitfall to assiduously avoid in conducting performance work. The client needs to know that you both are attuned to their loss of true self and are committed to address it in the work together. Although the presenting problem is behavioral and the ultimate outcome of the treatment will be assessed in these terms, the behavior has to be reintegrated into the self-experience. The question, "what does my performance mean to me?" naturally flows to the larger ones, "who am I?" and, "what do I want out of my life?"

7. As with all EMDR work; maximal education of the client of the process is essential. They need to be apprised that exploration and work with their personal and performance history will be essential. They also need to understand and agree to the degree of personal and affective exposure (to themselves and you) that may be needed to shift the behavior.

8. In practice, the three most important things are follow-up, and more follow-up. Mo matter what kind of shift or reprocessing goes on in session, it is no guarantee of improvement in performance. The follow up-session(s) gives the chance to see what has shifted and what hasn't. This provides the opportunity to install the positive changes (a reality template similar to the positive cognition). The remaining negative experiences can then be processed more narrowly. Hopefully, as sessions proceed, the positive experiences will widen and the negative will attenuate. Opportunities for in vivo work can also be valuable as the process develops. There can be value in working simultaneously with two parallel targets and protocols, one present day and behavioral, the other historical and underpinning the performance inhibition.

Back and forth movement between these protocols in one or a number of sessions will oftentimes accomplish synergistic movement in each.

9. Always remember that the goal, unless changed by mutual consent, is behavioral improvement as defined by the performer. They need to be guided and supported to determine when they have satisfactorily met the goal, even if more personal work remains to be accomplished.

*The neurological processes observable following a traumatic event appear parallel to those of a performer or athlete suffering from performance anxiety, creative blocks and loss of confidence. Accordingly, EMDR tends to reprocess and resolve these performance situations in the same rapid, effective manner it helps an individual move on from a traumatic experience. EMDR is also effective in releasing and resolving the ubiquitous stress experienced by corporate executives, as well as enhancing their decision-making abilities. EMDR is also helpful in containing the anxiety that often precedes a significant medical procedure, and has been used to maintain relaxation during surgery performed under local anesthesia. An athlete or performer recovering from injury or surgery frequently will suffer from fear of reinjury and loss of confidence in the efficacy of their body integrity. EMDR is effective in releasing the negative imagery and thinking which accompanies this recovery process.

How can you use EMDR ego state work with performance issues?

"Is the person in the performer or is the performer in the person?" All identity and ego state performance issues are subsumed under this question. Additionally, issues of performance are not usually seen in the larger context of development, traumatic life experiences, and self-perception. Performance, when framed primarily in terms of present tense sensory input and response, thought (beliefs) and behavior, is a limited concept. How we experience performance in the present is influenced by our ego states, especially the ones developed in early life. Positive or negative incorporations of our parents and caretakers were affected by how they responded to our early. These images transmute into ego states and are the foundation for our later performance experiences - both internal and external. When parents respond with positive mirroring (Kohut) such as excitement and reflections of, "look what Ellen did! She rolled over!" or "Billy, what a wonderful picture!" - early self-praising ego states tend to be initiated. However, when parents respond adversely or perhaps more damagingly by ignoring these early performances, both helpless, wounded as well as self critical, shaming and attacking ego states form. These traumas contribute to the development of performance perceptions of "I am bad" (shame development) or "I am invisible" (I don't exist). EMDR processing of present day performance anxiety often reveals the trauma of humiliation memories from school, especially elementary school - as well as the resulting wounded and self-attacking ego states.

Specific ego states exist within the athlete's, performer's and creative artist's identity. These are greatly determined by their performance experiences and history, both positive and negative. Common issues that influence the development of these ego states include: the individual's innate talents and proclivities, the dialectic between performing for oneself of for parents, coaches and teachers, as well as the capacity for adaptive obsessive/compulsive perseverance and dissociation from inordinate performance pressure and scrutiny.

EMDR ego states performance work is a specific application of the more general bilaterally enhanced separate-selves approach. Particular attention needs to be given to performance blocks and anxiety as well as how the presence or lack of resilience prevents or leads to extended performance inhibition (slumps). Self-attacking (critical, shaming, depriving) ego states need to be identified, understood and healed in terms of their woundedness, before addressing the victimized, vulnerable selves. Entities such as the competent performance self, the fun loving self, the peak performance self, the creative self, the balanced mind/body self and the spiritual self all can be marshaled to encourage, support and heal the suffering selves.

Performance anxiety is a dynamic process which is initiated by, as with social inhibition, the unconscious projection of distorted and self-attacking (critical, shaming, depriving) ego states onto the audience. This generates the false perception in the performer of failure and exposure of fraudulence that usually inhibits the individual's performance. A negative loop often develops which activates in the person both self-aggressive and terrified ego states, at times leading to the avoidance and withdrawal from performing. Treating this condition entails EMDR enhanced education regarding the process as well as the direct work with the panoply of ego states activated.

How do performance and creativity enhancement work differ?

Both performance enhancement and creativity enhancement are linked and overlapping however, clear differences exist. Performance enhancement entails the additional step of the shift from internal experience to specific behavioral tasks. Creativity enhancement is more internally oriented and flows more openly to external processes. Accordingly, it can be less difficult to work with unblocking creativity than moving inhibited performance. For example, writer's block can be at times reduced or dissolved simply by targeting the experiential and historical aspects of the blockage. This may or may not open up other channels that need to be processed. The positive to be installed can be the sensorial memory experience of flowing creatively. This unblocking leads to an opening up and flowing must lead to specific improvements in behavioral task functioning, which is in essence a focusing or narrowing down. For instance, a baseball player who feels more relaxed and confident at the plate has to be able to improve in his/her ability to perform the mechanics of connecting on the sweet spot of the bat with a spinning, moving orb approaching at in excess of 90 mph. Being in a state of flow means little unless the specific task can be performed with greater efficiency and reliability. This can be very difficult to attain, especially taking into account that those involved in high level performance are usually externally focused and out of touch or even dissociated from internal processes and flows naturally from the processing.

For over a year I have been working with actors, who are wonderful responders to EMDR. Much of their training and exercises are parallel to the EMDR process. They all have significant issues with feeling not good enough and fraudulent with considerable trauma in their backgrounds. Acting is both deeply creative and internal as well as external and performance oriented. I have also worked with writers, concert and rock musicians, graphic artists and professional athletes. Despite how highly effective EMDR is with these people, the performance world is an extremely difficult market to break into. You may be selling gold for the price of silver with no takers while those selling brass for the price of gold may have many flocking to them. If you enter into this field you must have supreme perseverance. Remember, perseverance is an achingly long race, although not a marathon. There is no finishing point and the winners are those who are still running while all others have dropped out.

What are some self-use EMDR techniques?

I use self-EMDR frequently in a variety of situations. It is amazing in helping retrieve information that slips your mind or is on the tip of your tongue. My son (15) uses it when taking tests and not sure which answer to choose. I also use it for relief of body stress, emotional distress and to foster my insight. I also have my clients use it, with my CDs and tapes or right on the spot - alternating finger of fist squeezing. This is similar to going for a walk to sort out your thoughts.

How have you used EMDR with actors?

Of all of the performance and creativity enhancement applications of EMDR, the most remarkable I have encountered is for acting. I have developed and implemented protocols for EMDR Acting Coaching (EAC). This technique is aimed at helping the actor to quickly reduce or eliminate performance and audition anxiety, explore characters in greater depth and texture and perform on stage with increased spontaneity and confidence. EAC blends traditional acting coaching techniques with a structured psychological approach accelerated by left/right brain hemisphere stimulation. The results have been dramatic (no pun intended).

Here is an example of EAC in action. In visualizing their role, the actor identifies their negative thoughts, anxiety and where they are held in the body. This is cleared with left/right tones, touch or eye movements. The actor is then guided to explore in their mind the profound events that have shaped the character's life. They are processed in with the same left/right which quickly and deeply bring these experiences to emotional life for the actor. The result is an almost startling power and newness that spontaneously emerges onstage.

Q & A on EMDR Performance Enhancement with golf:

Question: I am doing a presentation on peak performance in golf. During that presentation, I want to introduce my program and the types of coaching tools I have.

Answer: Perhaps you can give me an impression of your program for golf and any questions you have about performance issues. Have you heard of the "yips"? That is a lock-up or shaky reaction that causes golfers to miss short putts, lose their confidence, and get caught in a negative cycle they can't break out of, sometimes for years! The great Ben Hogan was known for chronically suffering from the yips. I think it has an OCD/panic like component and it would be interesting to study the larger clinical picture in which it is found. EMDR can be very helpful with this although oftentimes one has to go back to earlier developmental and trauma history for targets and resolution. Usually the underpinning is fear of failure or fear of success/guilt/masochism.

It is also interesting to take a history of the golfer. How old were they when they took up the game? Did they do it for themselves or for parents or others? What has been their history of skill development and appreciation and joy of the game? What has been their experience with lessons, tournaments, competition, gambling on the game or playing as an adjunct for business? What are female vs. male issues with golf? Issues of age, physical condition, emotional condition, concentration, learning. What are the golfer's strong and weak points: short game, long game, on the green, consistency? Is the first tee experience different than the fifth of the 14th?

Question: I agree that historical information is important and I get that information in the first session. I had heard of the "yips" per say, but I understand it conceptually.

Answer: Better learn the term because it is a biggie with golfers.

Question: You mentioned in vivo treatment is necessary and I would like to hear more about that.

Answer: It's pretty simple. With a client you have worked with in office, the opportunities for doing right on the spot - processing out of the negative and processing in of the positive are direct and powerful. For example, at the first hole or driving range, ask your client what they are thinking - how they are feeling emotionally and physically. If possible, have them process any negatives down to a zero SUDS. Then guide them to the positive (entailing the five steps) and install it. The client then takes the shot and you again process in the positive and out the negative. Repeat throughout retries or continuing on course. After completing the course, sit down and reprocess the entire experience. Remember - as EMDR therapists - we deal with performance issues with all of our clients - every day.

How do you treat fear of flying with EMDR?

In treating fear of flying, you initially need to assess if it exists as a discrete phobia or part of an overarching anxiety or panic disorder. If the phobia is discrete, it will be easier to process out. Your diagnostic assessment should include an extensive personal history that addresses the following questions: Does the client have any other phobias (especially driving phobias)? When did the fear start? Is the fear connected to a traumatic incident, especially one associated to flying? Is it symbolic of something? Did either of the parents of the client expose the client to an anxiety condition, especially fear of flying?

You can set up the protocol building from either the client's frightening mental imagery, a resonant memory or a negative cognition (we're going to crash, I'm definitely going to die, I can't survive without being in control) which emanates from the phobia.

While processing, be especially cognizant of the client's somatic experience. If you can fully clear the body sensations - you may have accomplished most or all of the reprocessing necessary. If the body sensations continue fluxing (changing in location, quality or image), without processing out, there is a possibility the client has an underlying panic disorder - which is of course more difficult to resolve.

Assuming you can reduce the SUDS down to a solid zero, you may then deepen the effect with an inoculation process combining EMDR and flooding. Work up together an imagined flying scenario which is frightening enough (i.e. extended turbulence described graphically) to re-elevate the SUDS level to a 5 or greater, build a protocol around it and again, process it down to a zero. Subsequently develop increasingly terrifying scenarios, i.e. a drop of 15 seconds or two engines going on fire. Continue the exercise until no imagined scenarios raise any charge. You can then install the positive future template of imagining a flight from waiting to board until deplaning with a sense of calm and control.

Of course, none of this has any value unless, as in all performance work, the client has a chance to perform the task in vivo. A follow-up session is scheduled to assess and install any gains accomplished and to more narrowly focus any remaining negative aspects of the experience. A trip to the airport is an easy exposure; a planned flight is the big challenge that holds the opportunity for full resolution. This can be a short shuttle run or a flight as part of a pleasure or business flight.

It is very important that the client be taught EMDR self stimulation - such as moving eyes between two spots on the wall, bilateral knee tapping or finger pressing, or use of equipment or CDs and tapes. This can provide anxiety control before and during flight (especially take off) and can be a very effective adjunct to the office treatment.

I have treated many who suffer from fear of flying, including two who were involved in plane drops of between 10 and 20 seconds with chaos and injuries on the plane. Usually a full or close to complete resolution of the phobia has been accomplished. The few exceptions have been clients with a significant panic disorder, a dissociative disorder or some hidden agenda that powerfully rewards not flying.

Q & A on stage fright (using Parallel Protocols):

Question: A Clinical question I have had with a very gifted 25 year old female violinist with a tremendous stage fright, who has an appointment next week asking for EMDR treatment. Do you have any kind of experience with this combination?

Answer: Your client's situation may be anything from basic to the most complex. The key thing is to determine whether this is a compartmentalized anxiety or part of a larger anxiety or panic condition. The first is much easier to resolve. Take a performance history - when the anxiety started, when it has been at its worst etc. I recommend using parallel protocols, starting with the current performance anxiety situation and then take the N.C. and ask her what incident from earlier in life, preferably from childhood, comes to mind and then build a protocol with that. Start by processing the earlier protocol but switching over to the recent one when shifts seems to happen. Just the process alone of setting up the two protocols will reveal a lot to you and the client.

Give the Performance of Your Life: Going from Stage Fright to High Light with EMDR: (an example of a marketing write-up on EMDR Performance Enhancement for audition anxiety)

Imagine this scenario, although it may not be much of a challenge to do so. You are awaiting an important audition that means the world to you. Slowly anxiety and self-doubt creep in like fog rolling in off the ocean. Your head feels like it is filled with helium, a fist of unknown origin grabs and twists your stomach and an electrical feeling courses through your body as if your ears were attached by jumper cables to a Sears DieHard. You can't escape the thoughts, "I'm not good enough," "I'm a fake; they'll see right through me," "I'm going to blow it," "Why am I putting myself through this humiliation and torture? Maybe I should leave." Your fingers now feel as if they are covered with ever thickening molasses and you know that doom is imminent. When you are called in you walk self consciously across the stage anticipating a loss of balance leading to a swan dive into the orchestra pit. "At least then I could slink away on my hands and knees unnoticed, never to be seen again." You sit down and look out at the blank, bloodless faces of those who will evaluate your performance and think, "They haven't heard a note so why are they thinking I stink like a week old catfish?" Although your fears don't materialize and the stage ceased feeling like the tilting deck of the Titanic, you are frustrated by the awareness that your anticipatory anxiety not only blocked your performing to your potential but also hurt like hell. Have you also ever, in an important orchestra performance, played an off beat or sour note that echoed through the hall like a bull moose call in mating season? To make things worse that sound stays with you for days like an ambulance is following you all your waking hours with its siren wailing. Going to sleep provides no escape as every time you close your eyes in bed you see the conductor's cruel laser stare that says to you, "I detest your incompetence. Die, fool!"

Remarkably there has been a recent breakthrough that is both spectacular and simple named EMDR (Eye Movement Desensitization and Reprocessing). Nothing out there is close to EMDR when it comes to controlling or even eliminating these irrational, distorted anticipatory fears. The technique is equally effective in helping you to let go and move on following either real or perceived failure. EMDR is also a powerful tool when used to reinforce and enhance the imagery, thoughts, feelings and sensory experiences associated with positive performance.

EMDR obtains its effect by alternating activation of the left and right hemispheres of the brain. This is accomplished by inducing left/right eye movements, touch or auditory stimulation. The individual starts by holding in mind simultaneously either a negative or positive 'freeze-frame' image, the associated self-belief together with the accompanying emotions. This ultimately leads them to process out the negative or process in the positive experience. As this procedure activates the neurological system the positive changes are almost always permanent. Of course with claims as bold as ours it is not only acceptable to be skeptical, it is wise and prudent. To be believed or even understood – EMDR has to be experienced. We have helped hundreds to benefit from this amazing process and we hope you are intrigued to give it a try. We are convinced that you will consider it a godsend!

Transitions - Associations of the Heart and Mind (A poem about the EMDR experience written while listening to Bio*Lateral*)

Part One
The mind is always in motion,
Thoughts skipping and sliding.
Some threads are visible
Some lie deeply buried in darkness.
Some crawl slowly by,
Others flash through or spring from nowhere.
Shadows shift in the twinkly twilight
And the dazy dawn.
Trauma skulks silently.

Music plays its key,
Time tags of the inside ears
Reposing senses and feelings.
The body is a tuning fork
Humming to harmonic time travel.
From now to then and back again.
Tones rouse drowsing memories
Long ago "forgotten."
Reawakened and finding new meaning.

Step into the car.
Flick on the radio.
Experience the transitions,
Associations of the heart and mind.

Part Two
As one journey ends
Another begins.
Exit the mind's freeway
And gently decelerate.
Glance into the rearview mirror.
Rememberances of things past
Are closer than they appear.

Associations of the heart and mind
Will continue unguided
By musical intermezzo,
As unconscious trains of thought
Traverse their unfolding tracks.
These subways of double helix
And loop the loop passages.

Remain open and alert
For those who listen to their
Transitions, associations of the heart and mind,
Receive the gift of creativity, wisdom and insight.

Part Six - Instructions for the use of Bio*Lateral* sound recordings

It is important to be cognizant that transitioning from eye movements to bilateral auditory stimulation for EMDR is a significant paradigm shift. If you have only used hand or finger movements, you may feel some confusion as well as loss of direct involvement with the client. This may feel uncomfortable at first although the benefits to you of less wear and tear on your shoulder, the ability to observe and take notes during processing will become apparent with time. The client will need to acclimate to the shift as well. Some will enjoy the sound immediately, others with difficulties in adaptability may need time to adjust to the change in approach. Try Bio*Lateral* with a new client and watch for their response - they require no adjustment.

Bio*Lateral* tapes and CDs were conceptualized to provide left/right auditory stimulation integrated into soothing music or sound. The purpose of this synthesis is to possibly lessen the intensity of client distress and abreaction. The sound can be like a safe place that is experienced simultaneously with the bilateral stimulation (some clients have stated this directly). As a result, processing may appear gentler or even obscure or distract ones awareness of the actual processing that is generated.

1. Trouble-shooting: What do you do if client reports, "nothing is happening," or "my mind went blank," or "I just relaxed"? Check things out just as you would in any EMDR situation using eye movements. Ask questions like, "You started with the image, emotions, body sensations, where did you go next? This may reveal that there was processing that went unnoticed. Keep in mind how many clients, when you first introduced to EMDR, struggled in acclimating during first few series of sets. Some may have needed longer sets before processing was activated. Some clients reported comments like, "nothing happened", or, "this feels silly", or "I'm afraid this won't work for me"? When this happened did you assume that EMDR wouldn't work for them or did you reassure or educate them and as they continued and got past their initial reaction and began to

process? It often works the same way with the introduction of auditory stimulation where some clients need to be guided past the initial awkwardness or need for education as far as what to expect.

2. What do I do if a client reports a loss of focus? As you know, any target is just a jumping off place and moving quickly to something else may be rapid, comfortable processing. Ask where the clients go when they report losing focus? If you bring them back to target has any discernible shift occurred in image or SUDS level? Any questions about lack of focus or relaxation can be addressed by having the client raise their level of distress before putting on the headphones, closing their eyes, bringing up the image and repeating the NC to themselves a few times.

3. What volume do I use? A louder volume tends to attract the attention of the client to the music or sound or away from the processing or awareness of it. I usually recommend the client listening at the lowest audible level. Imagine if you did eye movements so fast with constantly changing patterns or hand taps hard and fast; would the client be distracted by the intensity of the stimulation and have trouble processing? The human brain appears to be activated by the rhythm, not the volume. Any slight vibration of the eardrums will activate the opposite side of the brain, so don't be concerned about a low volume not working. Please check the working condition and volume of the sound, as well as the bilaterality of the tones before handing the headset to the client. Before you proceed, make sure the client can hear both tones delivered left and right. Although the lowest audible volume is recommended, the client has the option of increasing the volume. Those with any hearing impairment should especially be asked if they are hearing the tones out of both headphones.

4. How do I determine how long the sets should be? As a rule, sets tend to run longer with Bio*Lateral* than with eye movements. Start with a twenty-second set and gradually increase it from there, unless the client is highly dissociative. An advantage of the using the tapes is that clients can go for much longer sets (I have some experienced clients who will go for up to 2 to 5

minutes - getting into some very deep processing). Many experienced clients can learn to determine when to end the sets themselves, with you retaining the option to step in when you deem it appropriate.

5. What do I do if a client reports that they are listening to music? If the volume is high, have the client lower it. If the volume is low, tell them to keep going without concern and wait for thoughts to come to them. If you believe in it and convey confidence, they probably will as well. The opposite is also often true. Imagine you were teaching someone to drive and they made two incorrect moves (not dangerous). Would you pull them out of the driver's seat assuming they could never learn how? Missed opportunities result from jumping to conclusions and acting precipitously.

6. Further instructions for use of Bio*Lateral* tapes and CD: Please follow the 8 step preparation and procedure outlined in Dr. Francine Shapiro's 1995 textbook, "EMDR: Basic Principles, Protocols and Procedures," including use of DES with any clients showing any indications of dissociation, as well as installation of safe place.

The left/right aural tones produce bilateral stimulation and eliminate the need for eye movement (however clients may at times spontaneously move their eyes). Clients can choose to process with their eyes open or closed. Please note that eyes closed processing may differ from that with eyes open.

*Please be cognizant that processing with closed eyes may foster a dissociative response. If any adverse response such as severe dissociation or decompensation occurs at any point in the process, please discontinue by instructing the client to immediately remove the headphones. Accordingly, you should not use Bio*Lateral* with clients whom you suspect are highly dissociative, who have scored high on the DES or other rating scales or who have responded with high levels of dissociation to eye movements.

The tapes allow each set to continue as long as you or the client chooses. Sets can last for many minutes and may contain 100s or even 1,000s of repetitions. Please use shorter sets in the beginning until you have a sense of how your client is responding and keep track during longer sets to ensure that your client does not become overly dissociative or ungrounded. It is best to interrupt sets by removing the headphones, as opposed to turning the tape or CD player off and on.

No counting is necessary. Many therapists have reported that clients experienced with EMDR are often better able to determine the length of a set themselves as they are witnessing the processing "from the inside."However, the client should be instructed that the therapist retains the option of deciding to interrupt the set for any clinical reasons they ascertain.

Try having your client listen to Bio*Lateral* throughout the session, even when dialoguing with the therapist between sets. Also try using Bio*Lateral* during a non-EMDR session and determine at the end with the client if they experienced a difference.

With clients who respond well in session and are not unstable or dissociative, consider having them use Bio*Lateral* in between sessions to reduce insomnia, agitation, panic attacks, somatic distress and body pain and with urges (food, cigarettes, drugs) and compulsive behavior control. If this aspect is used, it is essential to instruct the client to immediately remove the headphones and interrupt the process if any adverse or intensely abreactive response occurs.

*It is recommended that you personally evaluate the effectiveness of Bio*Lateral* yourself before using with clients. Sit in a quiet place and think of something that is bothering you at that moment. Develop your own protocol, take a SUDS level and follow your associations. Then, observe the nature of your processing and occasionally return to target and retake the SUDS. Be especially aware of changes in body sensations.

More Books about EMDR:

Emotional Healing at Warp Speed: The Power of EMDR, by David Grand, Ph.D.

Brainspotting, by David Grand, Ph.D. Paperback and Kindle/E-book.

This is Your Brain on Sports, by David Grand, Ph.D. Paperback and Kindle/E-book.

Healing the Folks Who Live Inside: How EMDR Can Heal Our Inner Gallery of Roles, by Esly Regina Carvalho, Ph.D. Paperback and Kindle/E-book

Getting Past Your Past, by Francine Shapiro, Ph.D. Paperback and Kindle/E-book

EMDR: The Breakthrough "Eye Movement" Therapy for Overcoming, Anxiety, Stress and Trauma, by Francine Shapiro and Margaret Forrest. Paperback and Kindle/E-book

Handbook of EMDR and Family Therapy Processes, Francine Shapiro. Paperback.

EMDR: Basic Principles, Protocols and Procedures, by Francine Shapiro. Hardcover.

A Therapists Guide to EMDR: Tools and Techniques for Successful Treatment, by Laurel Parnell. Paperback.

EMDR Therapy and Adjunct Approaches with Children, by Ana Gomez. Paperback.

EMDR in the Treatment of Adults Abused as Children, Laurell Parnell. Paperback.

EMDR as an Integrative Psychotherapy Approach, Francine Shapiro. Hardcover.

Small Wonders: Healing Childhood Trauma with EMDR, Joan Lovett. Hardcover.

If you liked this book, we would appreciate a review on Amazon about it, so that others can benefit from your comments.

References - Diagnosis, Treatment and Ego States

- Berne, E. (1963). Structure and dynamics of organizations and groups. New York: The Grove Press.
- Blanck, G. and Blanck, R. (174). Ego psychology: theory and practice, New York: Columbia Univ. Press.
- Bliss, E.L. (1981). Multiple personalities: A report of 14 cases with implications for schizophrenia. Archives of General Psychiatry, 37:1388-1397.
- Boor, M. (1982). The multiple personality epidemic: Additional cases and inferences regarding diagnosis, etiology, dynamics and treatment. Journal of Nervous and Mental Disease, 170:302-304.
- Braun, B.G. (1986). The BASK model of dissociation. Dissociation, 1, 4-24.
- Bromberg, P. (1994). "Speak! That I may see you", some reflections on dissociation, reality and psychoanalytic listening. Psychoanalytic dialogues, 4(4): 517-547.
- Bromberg, P. (1996). Standing in the spaces. Contemporary psychoanalysis, Vol. 32(4): 509-535.
- Brown, D.P. & Fromm, E. (1986). Hypnotherapy and hupnoanalysis. New Jersey: Lawrence Erlbaum.
- Crabtree, A. (1992). Dissociation and memory: A 200 perspective. Dissociation, 5(2), 150-154.
- Comstaock, C.M. (1991). The inner self helper and concepts of inner guidance: Historical antecedents, its role within dissociation, and clinical utilization. Dissociation, 4, 165-177.
- Coons, P.M. (1986). Child abuse and multiple personality disorder. Review of the literature and suggestions for treatment. Child Abuse and Neglect, 10, 455-462.
- Erskine, R. (1997). Theories and methods of an integrative transactional analysis: a volume of selected articles, San Francisco: The TA Press.Federn, P. (1928). Narcisism in the structure of the ego. Int. Journal of Psychoanalysis, 9, 401-419.
- Federn, P. (1932). The ego feeling in dreams. Psychoanalytic Quarterly, 1, 511-542.
- Federn, P. (1943). The psychoanalysis of psychosis. Psychiatric Quarterly, 17, 319, 246-257, 480-487.

- Fine, C.G. (1989). Treatment errors and iatrogenesis across therapeutic modalities in MPD and allied dissociative disorders. Dissociation, 2: 77-82.
- Fine, C.G. (1991). Treatment stabilization and crisis prevention: Pacing the therapy of the multiple personality disorder patient. Psychiatric Clinics of North America, 14, 661-676.
- Fine, C.G. (1993). A tactical integrationalist perspective on the treatment of multiple personality disorder, In R.P. Kluft & C.G.Fine (eds.), Clinical perspectives on multiple personality disorder (pp. 153-153). Washington, DC: American Psychiatric Press.
- Fine, C.G. (1994). Cognitive hypnotherapeutic interventions with patients with MPD. Journal of Cognitive Psychotherapy. An International Quarterly, 8.
- Fine, C.G. and Lazrove, S. (1997). The use of EMDR in patients with dissociative identity disorder. In press.
- Freud, S. (1919). Lines of advance in psycho-analytic therapy. Standard Edition, 17: p. 168. London: Hogarth Press.
- Freud, S. (1937). Analysis terminable and interminable. Standard Edition, 23: pp. 217-219. London: Hogarth Press.
- Herman, J.L. (1992) Trauma and recovery. New York: Basic Books.
- Hilgard, E. (1977). Divided consciousness: multiple controls in human thought and action. New York: Wiley Press, expanded edition.
- Janet, P. (1919). English edition: Psychological healing (2 vols.). New York; Macmillan, 1925. Reprint: Arena Press, New York, 1976.
- Kluft, R.P. (1982). Varieties of hypnotic interventions in the treatment of multiple personality. American Journal of Clinical Hypnosis, 24, 230-240.
- Kluft, R.P. (1984). Treatment of multiple personality disorder. A study of 33 cases. Psychiatric Clinics of North America, 7, 9-29.
- Kluft, R.P. (1986). Personality unification in multiple personality disorder: A follow-up study. In B.G.Braun (Ed.) Treatment of multiple personality disorder. Washington, DC:

American Psychiatric Press, (pp. 29-60).

- Kluft, R.P. (1988). An update on multiple personality disorder. Hospital and Community Psychiatry, 38, 363-373.
- Kluft, R.P. (1988). On treating the older patient with multiple personality disorder: "Race against time" or "Make haste slowly?" American Journal of Clinical Hypnosis, 30, 257-266.
- Kluft, R.P. (1988). Editorial: Today's therapeutic pluralism. Dissociation, 1, 1-2.
- Kluft, R.P. (1989). Playing for time: temporizing techniques in the treatment of multiple personality disorder. American Journal of Clinical Hypnosis, 32, 90-98.
- Kluft, R.P. (1990). Incest and subsequent revictimization: The case of therapist-patient sexual exploitation, with a description of the sitting duck syndrome. In R.P. Kluft, (Ed.), Incest related syndromes of adult psychopathology. Washington, DC: American Psychiatric Press, (pp. 263-287).
- Kluft, R.P. (1993a). Basic principles in conducting the psychotherapy of multiple personality disorders. In Kluft, R.P. & Fine, C.G. (eds.), Clinical perspectives on multiple personality disorder 1. Washington, DC: American Psychiatric Press, (pp. 19-50).
- Kluft, R.P. (1993b). Clinical approaches to the integration of personalities. In Kluft, R.P. & Fine, C.G. (eds.), Clinical perspectives on multiple personality disorder 1. Washington, DC: American Psychiatric Press, (pp. 101-133).
- Kluft, R.P. (1993c). Countertransference in treatment of MPD. In J.P. Wilson & J. Lindy (Eds.), Countertransference in the treatment of post-traumatic stress disorder. New York: Guilford Press, (pp. 121-151).
- LeDoux, J. (1996). The Emotional Brain. New York: Simon & Schuster.
- Nicosia, G.J. (1995). Eye movement desensitization and reprocessing is not hypnosis. Dissociation, 8, 69.
- Paulsen, S. (1995). Eye movement desensitization and reprocessing: Its cautious use in the dissociative disorders. DISSOCIATION, 8, 32-44.
- Reich, W. (1976). Character Analysis. New York: Farrar, Straus and Giroux.

- Reiser, M. (1994). Memory in Mind and Brain: What Dream Imagery Reveals. New Haven: Yale.
- Shapiro, F. (1989a). Efficacy of the eye movement desensitization procedure in the treatment of traumatic memories. Journal of Traumatic Stress Studies, 2, 199-223.
- Shapiro, F. (1989b). Eye movement desensitization: A new treatment for post-traumatic stress disorder. Journal of Behavior Therapy and Experimental Psychiatry, 20, 211-217.
- Shapiro, F. (1991). Eye movement desensitization & reprocessing procedure: From EMD to EM/R - A new treatment model for anxiety and related traumata. The Behavioral Therapist, 14, 133-135.
- Shapiro, F. (1995). Eye movement desensitization and reprocessing (EMDR). Basic principles, protocols, and procedures. Now York: The Guilford Press.
- van der Hart, O., Brown, P. & van der Kolk, B. A. (1989). Pierre Janet's treatment of post-traumatic stress. Journal of Traumatic Stress, 2, 379-395.
- van der Hart, O., & Brown, P. (1992). Abreaction re-evaluated. Dissociation, 5, 127-140.
- van der Hart, O., Steele, K., Boon, S., & Brown, P. (1993). The treatment of traumatic memories: Synthesis, realization, and integration. DISSOCIATION, 6, 162-180.
- van der Kolk, B.A., & van der Hart, O. (1991). The intrusive past: The flexibility of memory and the engraving of trauma. American Imago, 48, 425-454.
- van der Kolk, B.A., Fisler, R. (1995). Dissociation and the fragmentary nature of traumatic memories: Overview and exploratory study. Journal of Traumatic Stress, 9, 314-325.
- van der Kolk, B., McFarlane A., Weisaeth, L., Eds. (1996). Traumatic Stress. N.Y.: Guilford Press.
- Vaughan, K, Armstrong, M.S., Gold, R., O'Connor, N., Jenneke, W., & Terrier, N. (1994a). A trial of eye 15. movement desensitization compared to image habituation training and applied muscle relaxation in post-traumatic stress disorder. Journal of Behavioral Therapy and Experimental Psychiatry, 25, 283-291.
- Vaughan, K, Weiss, M., Gold, R., & Terrier, N. (1994b). Eye-

movement desensitization. Symptom change in post-traumatic stress disorder. British Journal of Psychiatry, 164, 633-541.

- Watkins, H. (1984). Ego-state theory and therapy. In Corsini, R., ed., Encyclopedia of Psychology, Vol. 1. New York: Wiley, (pp. 420-421).
- Watkins, J.G. (1971). The affect bridge: A hypnoanalytic technique. International Journal of Clinical and Experimental Hypnosis, 19, 21-27.
- Watkins, J.G. (1978). The therapeutic self, New York: Human Sciences Press.
- Watkins, J & Watkins, H. (1981). Ego-state therapy. In Corsini, R., ed., Handbook of innovative therapies. New York: Wiley, (pp.252-270).
- Watkins, J & Watkins, H. (1991). Hypnosis and ego-state therapy. In Keller, P. & Heyman, S., eds. Innovations in clinical practice: a source book, Vol. 10. Florida: Professional Resource Exchange.
- Watkins, J & Watkins, H. (1997). Ego states: theory and therapy, New York: W.W. Norton
- Wilson, S.A., Becker, LA, & Tinker, RH. (1995). Efficacy of eye movement desensitization and reprocessing (EMDR) treatment for psychologically traumatized individuals. Journal of Consulting and Clinical Psychology, 63, 928-937.

References - Performance Enhancement

- Cameron, J. (1997) The Artists Way. N.Y.
- Campbell, D. (1997) The Mozart Effect. New York: Avon Books.
- Edwards, B. (1989) Drawing on the Right Side of the Brain. New York: Putnam.
- Foster, S., Lendi, J. (1997) EMDR, Performance Enhancement for the Workplace. San Jose: Performance Enhancement Unlimited.
- Galway, T. (1981) The Inner Game of Golf. NY: Random House.
- Goleman, D. (1995) Emotional Intelligence. New York: Bantam Books.
- Jourdain, R. (1997) Music, The Brain and Ecstasy. New York: Morrow.
- Manfield, P. (1998) Extending EMDR, New York: W.W.Norton.
- Roberts, G. (1992) Motivation in Sports and Exercise. Champaign, IL: Human Kinetic Books.
- Shapiro, F. (1995) EMDR: Princípios Básicos, Protocolos e Procedimentos. Brasília: Editora Nova Temática.
- Ungerleider, S. (1996) Mental Training for Peak Performance. PA: Rodale Press.

www.ingramcontent.com/pod-product-compliance
Lightning Source LLC
LaVergne TN
LVHW050934080826
845145LV00004B/1255

* 9 7 8 0 6 1 5 8 7 9 3 9 0 *